Laura Huxley
Piero Ferrucci

Illustrated by Paola Ferrucci

THE CHILD OF YOUR DREAMS

The Child of Your Dreams

Laura Archera Huxley
Piero Ferrucci

Illustrated by
Paola Ferrucci

CompCare Publishers
2415 Annapolis Lane
Minneapolis, Minnesota 55441

Works by the same authors:

Piero Ferrucci:
What We May Be

Laura Huxley:
You Are Not the Target
This Timeless Moment
Between Heaven and Earth
Oneadayreason to Be Happy

Library of Congress Cataloging-in-Publication Data

10/00

Huxley, Laura Archera.
    The child of your dreams.

    Bibliography: p.
    1. Prenatal influences.   I. Ferrucci, Piero.
II. Title.
RG635.H89   1987   618.2′4   87-18203
ISBN 0-89638-110-2

Cover and interior design by Susan Rinek

Inquiries, orders, and catalog requests should be addressed to
CompCare Publishers, 2415 Annapolis Lane, Minneapolis, Minnesota 55441
Call toll-free 800/328-3330 (Minnesota residents 612/559-4800)

I have lived in the pursuit of a vision, both personal and social. Personal: to care for what is noble, for what is beautiful, for what is gentle; to allow moments of insight to give wisdom at more mundane times. Social: to see in imagination the society that is to be created, where individuals grow freely, and where hate and greed and envy die because there is nothing to nourish them. These things I believe, and the world, for all its horrors, has left me unshaken.

—Bertrand Russell

Contents

In this book we will meet the Possible Human: an embryo, a fetus, a baby, a child, an adult, in whom the existing potentialities for love, intelligence, and beauty are brought to full expression. Of course, this person may be female or male; in fact he, or she, is likely to be gifted with qualities traditionally ascribed to both sexes. In order to overcome the bias inherent in our language, when talking about the Possible Human, or any possible or real person, we will use the feminine and the masculine genders in alternate chapters.

Acknowledgments

The Child of Your Dreams was born on the second weekend of April 1978, assisted by inspired godfathers and godmothers—Al Huang, Jean Houston, Frederick Leboyer, Ashley Montagu, Ram Dass, Virginia Satir, John Vasconcellos—and by 1,300 caring and cheering people. The occasion was the inauguration of Our Ultimate Investment—an organization for the nurturing of the Possible Human. To all we gratefully acknowledge the love and intelligence with which the *Possible Human*—so baptized by Jean Houston—was and is supported.

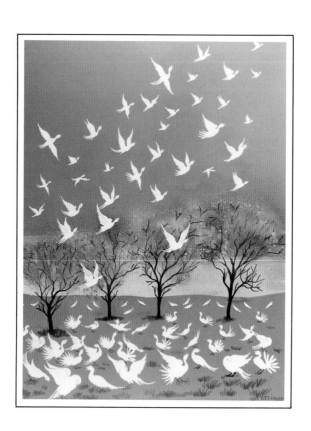

1 *The Child of Your Dreams*

*What a piece of work is a man! How noble in
reason! How infinite in faculty! In form and moving,
how express and admirable! In action, how like an
angel! In apprehension, how like a god! The beauty of
the world! The paragon of animals!*

—Shakespeare

Light. Undifferentiated, clear, blinding light. It is the light
of the future, so dazzling it is hard to sustain, because all
possibilities are in it. Then, out of the light, a form takes shape:
it is a form unknown, and yet so familiar. It has our shape, and
yet it is so alien. It attracts our attention—we want to see, we
want to know. We yearn to approach it. The form steps forward,
and from the unimaginable future it moves toward us. We can
clearly see its contours now. Imagine the smile, feel the complete
confidence. The light becomes less blinding, and we are beginning to realize whom we are facing. We know that it is one of
our kind. It is the Possible Human.

"How noble in reason! How infinite in faculty!". . .
There are few limits to what this creature can conceive or

imagine—the most abstract mathematical models, splendid forms and colors in painting and architecture, universal philosophical truths, melodies and rhythms that charm and inspire. He can challenge the secret workings of matter and delve into the mysteries of nature.

"In form and moving, how express and admirable!" . . . You remember the pleasure in seeing your favorite athlete, dancer, or mime; you are reminded of the beauty a versatile body can express, its grace and flexibility when moving, its refinement in gesture and shape. From chanting to dancing, from wrestling to making love, from running to diving to swimming, all movements may reveal the prodigious resourcefulness of the living organism.

"In action, how like an angel!" . . . What can a being do who is so endowed? What trace can he leave on the world he lives in? He acts swiftly and efficiently, touches countless people in beneficial ways; he explores unknown lands and spaces, reaches the highest mountains and the deepest abysses of the oceans; he heals the sick, helps the ignorant and the vulnerable; he teaches and inspires. Like the sun, he radiates light, warmth, life on those around him.

"The beauty of the world! The paragon of animals!" . . . Seeing human beings among horses and dolphins and birds, we realize that we originate from the symphony of nature—that we are, in fact, its highest and most refined achievement.

That is what this book is precisely about: the emergence of the person in whom all functions are brought to the maximum potential—and the opportunities we have of helping to create and nurture that ideal.

Research, reflection, experience, common sense—all show that an extremely sensitive period occurs during our lives when our physical and mental health, our attitude to the universe, our capacity to enjoy, to relate and to love can be either suffocated or allowed to blossom into full splendor. This crucial period starts long before birth, even before conception, and continues through conception, pregnancy, birth, and infancy. The extraordinary fact is that our destiny is decisively influenced during a time when we are, to all appearances, powerless and choiceless.

You, the adult reading this book now, have already gone through this sensitive period long ago. You may, however, participate in opening up wonderful opportunities for those who still are to enter it: unborn babies. As a potential or actual parent, you may choose to give birth to the child of your dreams. Thus, it may be your privilege and your duty to participate in the process of nurturing a person's potential—a process which in no way is the private domain of two parents alone, but is truly the Ultimate Investment which this tired, endangered, confused, magnificent humanity can lay its hope in.

But you may protest: "This is a hopeful endeavor to better the quality of the life of people in the future. But I have already gone through this sensitive period from conception to infancy, I have already crystallized in my grooves and become familiar with my scars and learned the dirty devices of the world. Yes, I am just a normal human being, not the possible human. If I ever participate in this adventure, it can only be as a witness, a helper perhaps, but no more. Those extraordinary possibilities you talk about have nothing to do with me."

Nothing, in fact, could be further from the truth. Through the years, as negative thoughts are repeated in our minds, many of us end up with a restricted or weakened self-image. And yet by the same gift of thinking we can extend the boundaries of the possible. In emergencies such as accidents of all sorts, natural catastrophes, war, and the like, ordinary human beings can perform extraordinary feats: they can show incredible physical strength, and they can be altruistic and heroic. During those dramatic instances their limited self-image is short-circuited, their latent powers are suddenly called into play. Why not try, then, to facilitate the use of these resources?

The Possible Human is within each one of us, whatever our age, creed, social position, talent, or state of health—open to what may be, always capable of trusting that something new and beautiful may happen. Yet, without this state of mind no change is possible.

Certainly, unconceived babies are on center stage. They, more than any others, may benefit from the suggestions and ideas here. But, as you will realize while reading on, within each of us there is a baby who needs to be protected and nurtured, who wants to come forward and live in what we feel and do. All that is beautiful and valuable in ourselves longs to be expressed, and yet so often, out of shyness, busyness, or forgetfulness, remains unborn. Are you willing to give this child within a chance?

Each chapter of this book presents several guided meditations designed to expand your consciousness of what a human being can be. You may want to just glance through them. If they hold any meaning for you, you could perhaps try them out and observe your reaction: the change in your self-image, the reverberations in your life. In any of these experiments, it's useful to take the attitude of the apprentice. In the world of subjective experience, change is the rule, not the exception. No meditation you repeat will give the same results; therefore if you give it a new try, you may be in for a surprise. As with muscle, you strengthen your inner faculties by using them. Finally, if you are a parent or parent-to-be, these meditations are of the greatest significance and usefulness.

Meet the Possible Human

Close your eyes, and take some time to put yourself fully at ease. Sit comfortably, eliminate all tensions, breathe deeply, slowly, and easily a few times.

Now become aware of your inner world, the world of feelings, images, thoughts. You don't have to do anything in particular with them now. Just be aware of them for a while, without judging or trying to change them.

Now imagine being in a dark tunnel. With all your senses perceive everything clearly and vividly. What you visualize is so real that you feel you are there yourself.

See the light at the end of the tunnel not too far from you.

While you walk in the dark, the light begins to grow brighter. You are proceeding toward it. As in a seed, the light contains infinite possibilities of beauty, compassion, and joy.

In this light you now recognize a point of condensed energy. It is a minuscule, fertilized human egg. You see the tremendous activity of cells dividing and taking the shape of a tiny embryo.

Gradually, the embryo grows. It is reminiscent of the ancient phases of our evolution. You watch with awe. Each stage is a new and surprising development.

You see this silent unfolding in the clearest of details, as if you had X-ray sight: the heart, so tiny yet, starts its vital task; as a galaxy of luminous points, countless cells are blossoming in the brain; the skeleton is taking shape; with exquisite precision the vital organs are developing; the eyes are becoming ready to see, the ears to hear; and, in looking at the little hands, you can almost feel their astonishing sensitivity. You see a miracle happening. You greet the newborn baby.

Now you see the baby growing into a child. He reaches out, starts to crawl, then the great change happens—he walks upright, and what an accomplishment that is! It is the beginning of a great adventure. His perceptions are becoming more accurate, his movements more purposeful. The child is now turning into an adolescent and then a fully developed adult. Millions of years of evolution, of learning, of accomplishments, are passing in a few instances in front of your inner eye.

For a few moments, meditate on what a piece of work, what a wonder, a human being is.

See this person reaching a further stage of evolution. Tremendous abilities and qualities are developed to their highest peak: love, intelligence, the exquisite capacity of creating beauty, the strength to dare, and the courage to challenge the unknown—all are brought to a full, wonderful flowering. You spend some time with this person, experience his or her presence. You become acquainted with the Possible Human.

And now you feel an affinity, perhaps recognize a likeness with this person. Then, lo and behold, you see that the Possible Human is, in fact, yourself! Coming from a faraway realm in the future stages of evolution, this person is yourself, the being that you can become.

And now you and the Possible Human fuse and become one and the same being. You are alone again now, but you have found your true Self. You feel in yourself the same love, the intelligence, the capacity of creating beauty, the strength to dare and the courage to challenge the unknown, which you have previously perceived in the Possible Human.

A Mozart sonata delights us with the contrast between a tragic movement and a joyful one; in a Greek temple the empty space gives meaning to the columns; a sunset spellbinds us with the clash between the sun's radiance and the large, shadowy clouds. There is no light without darkness. What makes our human adventure so compellingly fascinating is precisely *contrast*—the contrast between intelligence and ignorance, the struggle of beauty against ugliness, the ageless contest between tenderness and brutality. Who will win in the end? Even more relevant, who is going to win *now*, or the next day, or in the next few years?

We are all involved in this drama, or, if you will, in this dance. Nothing in it should be taken for granted, for intertwined with the creative potentialities are the possibilities of destructiveness, pain, and evil. With surprising rapidity and cunning, they branch out and are spread abroad. If you look deep into their origins, you see that they are never created out of nothing: the burglar who penetrates your home, the drug addict, the child abuser, the exalted warmonger, the religious zealot, and above all, the "normal neurotic" who is often in charge of the world we live in, are the results of negative chain reactions originating in the remote past.

All potentialities—beauty, intelligence, and love, as much as cruelty, dishonesty, and malice—exist in a newborn baby. In fact, we could say they are in the embryo, in the fertilized egg—

even in the fantasies and the intentions of two human beings who, desperately or serenely, skillfully or awkwardly, try to break out of their own solitude and love—or try to love—each other.

Once more, then, we come to those critical times:

—the time before conception, when a human being, not yet present in flesh and bones, already exists in the unfathomable levels of the possible;

—the time of conception, the most mysterious one, because even though we have full knowledge of it from the physical perspective, we can only fantasize what it may be from the standpoint of consciousness;

—the time of pregnancy, a period in which the blueprint of existence is prepared;

—the moment of birth, what may be the most dreadful shock of all, or the most loving and joyous beginning;

—the first days and months, when the relationship with the parents and the world is established.

These are the times in which the best seeds should be planted—seeds which at later times, even *much* later times in an individual's life, are most likely to grow strong and bear luxuriant fruits.

The good news is that if even a small part of today's knowledge on these matters were to be applied, a tremendous uplifting of the human condition would occur. The secret here lies in that subtle factor that distinguishes effective from ineffective education, and that is *timing*.

The greatest ideas lose much of their value if they are used when the best moment is past; and the most heartfelt affection will be received with infinitely greater benefit if it is expressed when it's most needed. This book contains no prescriptions which are beyond the bounds of each of us. Rather, it shows the wonders that even a tiny bit of goodwill and awareness can create when they happen at the right time.

One thing is certain: during the vulnerable formative period of life described, much is totally beyond our control, because so many forces—cosmic, biological, social, and personal—participate in the molding of a human being. On the other hand, much can be done to enhance the development of the future child.

Also, the most fundamental part of our adventure, the one that sets the mood and starts all future chain reactions, is the beginning. In life's beginning many things may happen that stimulate a human being's potential for good or for evil; much may happen that decides if a human being is going to fully live or merely survive.

The difference between *surviving* and *living* is fundamental. Surviving means having to fight one's way through life with diminished equipment, like fighting a battle with inadequate weapons. Such a person rarely experiences inner peace and the joy of living. In relationships he is never fully at ease with others. In using his mind, it's difficult to learn, remember facts and read with ease and pleasure. Physically, he falls victim to chronic fatigue and weakness. In the practical realm, simple daily operations become momentous tasks. For these people surviving turns one single day into a heroic saga—a saga that no one else will be able to fully comprehend. Occasional relief is hardly sufficient to enable the survivor to pull through, as he physically and mentally slouches onward through an impoverished life.

Compare surviving with being able to fully live—the condition of existing without destructive mechanisms, physical pain or insecurity. Above all, fully living is the situation where work and play become one; intelligence and imagination are used *at their peaks*; relationships are ever-renewing delights; each day is a source of new discoveries. What you are doing happens to be exactly what you like to do, and strength, confidence, and joy are the basis of all experience. Indeed there is pain too and there is ignorance, for these are inevitably a part of the human lot, but when they occur, one is able to learn from them and change. Walt Whitman splendidly described it all:

> In that condition the whole body is elevated to a state by others unknown—inwardly and outwardly illuminated, purified, made solid. Strong, yet buoyant. A singular charm, more than beauty, flickers out of, and over, the face— a curious transparency beams in the eyes, both in the iris and in the white—the temper partakes also . . . Sorrows and disappointments cease—there is no more borrowing trouble in advance. A man realizes the venerable myth—he is a god walking the earth, he sees new eligibilities, powers and beauties everywhere; he himself has a new eyesight and hearing. The play of the body in motion takes a previously unknown grace. Merely to move is then a happiness, a pleasure—to breathe, to see, is also. All the beforehand gratifications, drink, spirits, coffee, grease, stimulants, mixtures, late hours, luxuries, deeds of the night, seem as vexatious dreams, and now the awakening.

It is easy to change the direction of a stream at its source, a taoistic proverb tells us; but when the stream has become a mighty river, it is impossible to change its course. So it is with people. At the beginning, a human being is so very vulnerable and open to impression, and this may spell triumph or tragedy. What makes the difference? Of all the factors affecting us, one encompasses them all: it is our consciousness. The awareness with which a human being—present or future—is surrounded, the thoughts and the feelings it is nurtured with, the intentions that create it, the vision which gives it form and direction— these are the elements which affect its future development.

The Child of Your Dreams

With your eyes closed, relax and gradually let yourself find the place in you which is completely silent and still. Listen to the silence for a few moments until you become the silence.

Now vividly imagine yourself to be inside a sphere of golden light. You can feel it circulating in you, pervading you, breathing in you. This light is full of warmth and love: love that does not imprison but liberates; love that is not based on illusion, but on total awareness; love that helps each person become what he or she is meant to be.

Now, in this inner environment which you have created, imagine a world in which conception is conscious and responsible, pregnancy a time of tenderness, birth a moment of joy—a world in which babies and children are treated with kind-ness and intelligence, where humankind has learned to reproduce itself with awareness and love. Let images emerge of how this world could be, and also feelings, ideas, intuitions.

Imagine this society, where that which is most helpless receives care and tenderness, where the future is envisioned with intelligence. Think of how relationships would be different: a world without war, without diffidence and fear, where people could communicate with open hearts. Imagine this new age, in which all kinds of talents are celebrated and cultivated. And remember, in imagination everything is possible; therefore do not let any present skepticism undermine what you can envision.

Now imagine one of the future children from this world. Imagine that you are with this child, that he or she communicates with you, with words or silently, through the skin, as you hold it, or through the eyes. There is an intense flow of feeling between the two of you. Something beautiful, unnameable, happens—a contact that reaches deep down in you, behind all your defenses and armors, in the secret place where you are vulnerable, where you yourself are a child too.

Then with your own rhythm and timing, open your eyes and come back to everyday consciousness.

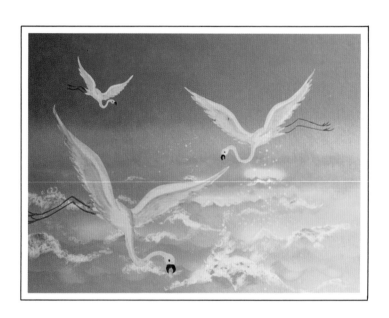

2 Prelude to Conception

He who hesitates is sometimes saved.

–James Thurber

Alone, you are in the middle of space, the open space of your life. You raise your eyes away from your day-to-day struggles and look all around you, near and far. Of the possible choices you see, some are alluring, others frightening. Some materialize near you with the reassuring contours of familiarity. Others, looming in distant landscapes, are yet enveloped by the mists of the unknown. Realistically, you remind yourself that some of these shapes are merely dreams. However, you also realize that even in the most trying of situations, even when time, money and other people's lives impose their pressures, you can retain some power in shaping your own existence.

Ever attentive, surveying a wide scene, you distinguish an increasing number of details. And now, look! The mists are gradually dissolving. You can see far into the depths of space and time. Your possibilities multiply, you get an impression of vastness, almost of infinity. So many things you may learn are emerging—people you could meet, places to explore, paths to tread, possible careers and interests, new traits and skills you can cultivate in yourself. Overwhelmed, you turn away; choices are anguishing, and you know that for anything you choose you also give up an infinity of other possibilities. Again you raise your eyes. The landscapes of your alternative universes look amazing now: there are people, ideas, unknown lands, all sorts of enticing shapes continually moving and shifting in colored, flashing whirlpools.

And now, in all of this dazzling array, something suddenly and powerfully attracts your attention. It is the face of a baby. It is your future baby. Her eyes, filled with innocence and the purest of joy, her sheer defenselessness, her funny sounds, her smile, her arms reaching toward you—they all evoke in you an overwhelming rush of tenderness. This is all so beautiful you forget all other choices. You are already embracing your baby. How could you leave her there alone, in the future, as a mere possibility? This is what you want—your whole nature is crying for it! You feel her tender skin, her hands playing with your face, her little cries of happiness, and the cleanliness of her breath, still pure as mountain air, playing on your cheek. You are embracing love itself.

You see her sleeping the deepest and most serene sleep under the heavens. If you are a woman, you are breastfeeding her. In that most archetypal of all activities, you are giving her the most natural and intimate of all nourishments. And you realize this is your baby—the baby who, body and soul, day after day, you created yourself. What a privilege! And what a temptation!

But wait! Don't lose all perspective yet. Look again—objectively and further into the future. Look at the whole picture: sleepless nights, a baby that cries and needs to be fed regularly when you would like to just rest and forget, a baby continuously and irrevocably present in your life. Not just for one hour, for play and fondling; not just for a pleasant afternoon of relaxation; not just for a day, as an exquisite gift of life; but day, after day, after day—and night, after night, after night. This little tyrant constantly demands attention. Perhaps you find yourself standing powerless in front of this little creature raging with a primordial energy that is almost frightening—and why, why is she crying so desperately? You are faced with chores and responsibilities that pile up with the rapidity of a nightmare. You would like to go to a movie, go for a walk, or visit friends. But you can't—or you can, but only if you make elaborate arrangements. You dream of being on your own, ah, the space, the delightful silence, the luxury of an empty afternoon. But it is impossible.

And now you look further into the future: the baby is growing up, it's kindergarten time, so off to school. She gives you wonderful satisfaction and comes up with those delightful expressions and ideas which only the innocent can invent. It's great to watch her learn something new every day, and visibly, miraculously grow in so many ways at once. She evokes tenderness and amusement in you, but sometimes she can turn into a little devil. It's time to go out, and "No, no, no, I won't put my shoes on." It's cold outside, and "No, no, no, I won't wear the coat." You have to eat if you want to grow and be strong, and "No, no, no, I don't want granola. I want chocolate ice cream." You are in the car and it's late, and "No, no, no, no, no, I am not going to sit in the baby seat. I want to drive the car." You are in the supermarket, and where has she gone now? Is she behind the beverages or the fruit? Or was she the one who knocked down a pile of cans?

Once again you look forward in time: this child is growing. She needs, as always, personal attention. Now she also needs to be followed in her schoolwork. More and more time and money are necessary to provide her with food, clothing, education, entertainment. She is becoming an adolescent—rebellious, unpleasant, aloof, temporarily a monster, as all respectable adolescents are bound to be. Your house is invaded by a gang of similar monsters, leaving a broad trail of soft drinks, loud music, disorder.

There are worries, too. The dark possibilities of accidents, violence, and drug addiction. "Not my child!" Yes, your child as well, possibly, for your child is no longer "yours" to guide and protect. With ever-increasing speed and intensity she is at the mercy of social forces beyond your control. Much can be done to prevent these evils, yet they still strike even the healthiest of families.

And what about your own wishes? Of course, as time goes on and you make your choices, your life, as anyone else's, becomes more structured and less open. Possibilities just snap closed, and you are pitilessly pinned down with the consequences of what you have chosen.

Naturally this is much more so when children are around. Upgrading your career . . . snap, it is not possible. You rightly want to give your child the attention and the time which is her inalienable right, or you would be gnawed by guilt.

Those evening courses on computers or cooking or flower arrangement . . . snap, by the end of the day, who has any energy left?

Your wish for a rich social life, travelling, meeting people . . . snap, snap. No more, too much money involved.

That peaceful time to be on your own, to read and learn a new language, devote yourself to a hobby, or, for heaven's sake, just do nothing . . . snap, snap, snap. Out of the question.

This scenario may seem much too dark to you. Perhaps the possibilities we have mentioned are sheer bliss to you: the piling up of laundry is for you like storing up a treasure; losing sight of your child in the supermarket becomes a comical game of hide-and-seek; everyday routine turns into a heavenly dance; and who cares about careers or travels when all you are interested in is the much more engaging and deeper adventure of caring for your loved ones? Both men and women are involved in this situation. You, the woman, may feel totally and specifically endowed by nature to be a mother. Many women feel diminished if they have to choose between family and career; you sense that you can juggle with both, or perhaps you are satisfied by mothering alone. You feel fulfilled in knowing that, through the care and education of your children, you will be engaged in shaping the world of tomorrow. And you, the man, are ready at least temporarily to forsake some of your ambitious projects, and create in your life, as the foremost priority, a wide and comfortable space in which, together with your family, you can be happy and peaceful. If this is so, fine— you know what you want.

But such an unambiguous outlook is rare. Most of us are fascinated by more than one possibility and do not see clearly the consequences of the choices we make. Anything we are bound to choose—mate, school, career, place to live—will shape our lives and make of us, gradually or abruptly, a new person, more inspired and vital or bitter and burned out. Any choice can be made in one of two main ways. It can be met with full awareness, or it can be unconscious, caused by a myriad of obscure sensations, feelings, instincts: "I don't know what made me take such a step . . . I don't know what came over me. . . ." A choice can be responsible or irresponsible. It may be the unthinking reaction of immediate self-gratification, or it may consider our own long-range aims and deeper satisfactions. A choice may be taken in a hurry with shallow breath or from a centered outlook in deep peace. There may even be no choice at all, but the relentless mechanism of compulsive behavior. Finally, a decision may be made in an atmosphere of resignation or of dreamy optimism—or, on the other hand, with a realistic trust in the potential of life.

All of these factors are going to affect not only the moment of choice but also the consequences of this choice during the years to come. Suppose your decision is about buying

a car. If it has been harried and haphazard, unpleasant consequences will possibly nag you with irritating insistence. Every
time you pay too much for gas consumption, hear that unpleasant squeak, or sign yet another check for increasing insurance,
you are reminded that there were better choices. A moment of
unawareness led you to unnecessary discomfort.

Be that as it may, a car is only a car. But think now of
deciding to have a son or daughter, a human being. By what
forces will this person be propelled into the universe?

There are many answers to this question. Statistics show
that one baby out of five in this country is born unwanted. Some
children are born because one of the two partners is trying to
"save the marriage" and hold a mate who is growing increasingly
distant. Some children are born because one or both parents
long for love, power, or a purpose in life. Perhaps the parent
needs an identity—to be "mother" or "father" gives a definite
positive image. In some situations, financial advantages and other
rights are received because of the child. Often a child is the
result of carelessness or of one drink too many, while others are
born out of sheer resignation—just because "it is the natural
thing to do," and social customs push us along predetermined
grooves. Other children are born because their parents need an
"experience no one should miss." Or because "after all these
girls, we need a boy."

Think of this person, at age two, or ten, or twenty, when
little by little it will dawn on her that she was born by chance;
or that, wanted in the first place, she has become the bitter
symbol of all that you had to give up; or, worse still, in a flash
of tragic awareness, that she was unwanted, the deepest of all
humiliations. Perhaps it won't come from anything you say
explicitly—but subtly, in your tone of voice, the way you look
at her or the substance of your everyday interaction. In contrast,
what atmosphere will surround the baby-child-person who has
been really wanted and chosen with a clear awareness of all

consequences—when the force that brought her into life has been a full, deep YES that came from the heart and mind? If this is the case, you will be able to look at your baby laughing, at your child playing or going to school, at your son or daughter confidently moving forward in the challenges of each day, and silently tell him or her, "Yes, I wanted you fully. I looked at all other possibilities life was offering, one by one, and then I chose you, because you are the very best and most beautiful one. I truly loved you, long before you were born."

There is an elegant and simple way of choosing. We can handle things at the source, not when they have solidified, not when we feel regrets and resentments, nor when we have to retrace our steps and pay for the consequences of mindless deeds. Being blurred by the urgency of physical desires, pretending to overlook future developments, allowing oneself to be enticed by the lure of false promises—this is not the way of mindful choice. Sometimes we dream of having children who will accomplish what we have failed to do or to enjoy what we missed. Can we, instead, be more objective and leave aside our needs and dreams for a moment? Then we will realize that children have their own being, with no need to replicate another's journey or represent anybody else's lineage.

Also, it would be helpful to keep in mind one basic factor: our society is now quite different from the time when we were children—whatever our age may be at present. The drastic decline in the extended family, the opening of greater opportunities for women, the technological explosion, social mobility, the relativity of values, the ever-increasing rate of change—these factors make our milieu the most complex of all social experiments, and probably the least emotionally secure of all environments for children to grow in.

Still, many powerful factors push us almost irresistibly towards having children: first of all, the ancestral urge of the species to perpetuate itself (and the species knows nothing about bills, careers, or divorces); secondly, the warm glow of tenderness—or the impelling urge of hormones, however we may want to phrase it; moreover, cultural pressures—of course everybody has children!

Finally, the trickiest and the most wondrous factor of all is the spontaneity of life. "Life is spontaneous," you say. "Trees grow without thinking; gazelles, eagles, and tigers reproduce themselves regardless of planned parenthood, according to the deepest animal instinct, survival. What else but cold intellectuality separates us from nature? The trouble is that we want to plan and control everything, instead of surrendering to the flow of events. Shouldn't we live, rather, as the lilies of the field?"

Certainly we all are awed by the beauty and miraculous ease with which nature takes its course. We all have experienced that same grace in ourselves, if only for a passing moment, and long to participate in it again. Touched by nostalgia for a lost paradise, we wish to find once more the courage to fully trust in the natural order without fear or reservation. But that trust is immensely different from mere blind impulse. Impulse may bring about the pain of unwanted children who, as all evidence shows, are more likely to be battered, less likely to be law-abiding, or will just be unhealthy and unhappy. Trust makes full use of our most precious achievements: the respect and love which foresee the consequences of our actions; the creative imagination that makes our life a work of art; the strength to look at things objectively; the peace that allows us to be fully behind our choices. Only this deep trust, born of our entire being, can make us feel again one with the lilies of the field and the whole of nature.

Prelude to Conception

The thoughts presented here as the Prelude to Conception must be the concern of anyone even vaguely considering the possibility of conceiving a child. If that includes you, you may want to try the following exercise. Compared with other meditations you can find in this book, it will be rather different, longer, and perhaps more difficult. However, you are now faced with an immensely important choice—to have or not to have a child. A small amount of effort and concentration now can save you, your partner, and the child much unexpected difficulty, complications, suffering and conflicts at a later time.

The exercise you are presented with has the purpose of envisioning clearly and in detail what it would be like for you to raise a child. This task entails several factors, and you will be guided through each of them. Two qualities are essential in doing this work: sincerity with yourself and precision.

Although the following looks like a questionnaire, it is not. You are not asked to simply read these questions and briefly answer them. Rather, you have to stop at each one of them, visualize the situation involved vividly and in detail, and imagine yourself fully involved in it. In all likelihood, you will have to spend quite a while on each question, so it will probably take more than one session to complete the exercise. Remember, if you feel the temptation to move quickly on, please resist. Some questions may raise problems and unpleasant circumstances, and your mind may perform all kinds of tricks to persuade you to skip what you need most to consider.

Before starting each session, make sure you have ample time for yourself, that no pressures will disturb or distract you. Have pencil and paper handy if you want to take notes. You can use colored pencil and also draw your answer. (It does not matter in the least whether you know how to draw or not.) Begin with some deep breathing and centering, then go on to the first group of questions:

Does having and raising a child fit with the lifestyle I want?

1. What do I want out of life for myself? What do I think is important?

2. Could I handle a child and a job at the same time? Would I have time and energy for both?

3. Would I be ready to give up the freedom to do what I want to do, when I want to do it?

4. Would I be willing to cut back my social life and spend more time at home? Would I miss free time and privacy?

5. Can I afford to support a child? Do I know how much it takes to raise a child?

6. Do I want to raise a child in the neighborhood where I live now? Would I be willing and able to move?

7. How would a child interfere with my growth and development?

8. Would a child change my educational plans? Do I have the energy to go to school and raise a child at the same time?

9. Am I willing to give the most creative part of my life—AT LEAST EIGHTEEN YEARS—to being responsible for a child? And spend a large portion of my life being concerned about my child's well-being?

How will I benefit by having a child?

1. Do I like doing things with children? Do I enjoy activities that children can do?

2. Would I want a child to be like me?

3. Would I try to pass on to my child my ideas and values? What if my child's ideas and values turn out to be different from mine?

4. Would I want my child to achieve things that I wish I had, but didn't?

5. Would I expect my child to keep me from being lonely in my old age? Do I do that for my parents? Do my parents do that for their parents?

6. Do I want a boy or a girl child? What if I don't get what I want?

7. Would having a child show others how mature I am?

8. Will I prove I am a man or a woman by having a child?

9. Do I expect my child to make my life happy?

What do I need to know about raising a child?

1. Do I like children? When I'm around children for a while, what do I think or feel about having one around all the time?

2. Do I enjoy teaching others?

3. Is it easy for me to tell other people what I want, or need, or what I expect of them?

4. Do I want to give a child the love he needs? Is loving easy for me?

5. Am I patient enough to deal with the noise and the confusion and the twenty-four-hour-a-day responsibility? What kind of time and space do I need for myself?

6. What do I do when I get angry or upset? Would I take things out on my child if I lost my temper?

7. What does discipline mean to me? What does freedom, or setting limits, or giving space mean? What is being too strict, or not strict enough? Would I want a perfect child?

8. How do I get along with my parents? What will I do to avoid the mistakes my parents made?

9. Would I take care of my child's health and safety? How do I take care of my own?*

> *Reread this questionnaire at each birthday. If your resolution is* no, I will not have a child—*or at least not for now—think about all the space, the freedom, the opportunities you have so easily created for yourself. And if your answer is* yes, *oh what a Great Story this is going to be, charged with more suspense than a mystery, more adventure than an epic, and hopefully more laughter than the most delightful comedy!*
>
> *Yes, this is the story of your child—the child of your dreams. She is beginning now in the earnestness with which you look inside yourself. One day many years from now, you and your child will be going for a walk on a sunny day, or coming back home in the evening, or maybe it will be goodnight time, and something in the atmosphere will tell you, she is ready. This is the moment to let her know. You will feel a very special tenderness, perhaps a touch of awe. Then you will let her know. You will tell her the Great Story: how*

*Reprinted with permission from "Am I Parent Material?" Network Publications, a division of ETR Associates, Santa Cruz, CA.

long before she came into being you thought and prepared yourself for her.

You will tell her about the certainty you felt when you conceived her—that deep certainty you could only have reached after a strenuous and honest look within yourself.

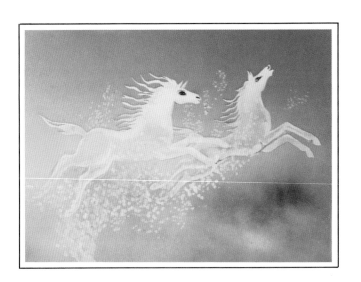

3 *Conscious Conception*

*The first step which we make in the world is the
one on which depends the rest of our days.*

– Voltaire

Can you imagine the Greatest Explosion That Ever Took
Place? Astronomers tell us that our universe started with a Big
Bang, "an explosion which occurred simultaneously everywhere, filling all space from the beginning, with every particle
of matter rushing apart from every other particle." The temper-
ature was a hundred thousand million degrees and the universe
was filled with light. Only much, much later did it differentiate
into galaxies and stars.

Another explosion much closer in time and space to you
was just as momentous: it took place when a sperm and an egg
came together and created you. This event is usually not
described in such terms in the average biology textbook.
However, when regressed to the moment of their own conceptions, a number of individuals report this experience as a joyous
burst of the exultant fireworks of life. Moreover, just as the echo
of the explosion which initiated the universe reverberated
throughout the universe as a background noise, likewise the
quality of that moment of conception is still echoing in your

personal universe. And your cells, your bodily structure, your nervous system, the secret corridors of your brain, the blood flow and the very breath of life still resonate with your own initial explosion.

Surely, if you just try to remember the very beginning of yourself, it feels like reaching back in the dark cloud of unconsciousness. You grope in obscurity, and yet you vaguely feel that you came from a different realm, from elsewhere:

> *The soul that rises with us, our life's Star,*
> *Hath had elsewhere its setting,*
> *and cometh from afar.*
> *– Wordsworth*

Wordsworth's lines are beautiful, but they generate questions for the mind to struggle with. Is there an individual soul? Where does it come from? Were we conscious before birth? Are we ultimately a Consciousness transcending time and space? Had the circumstances in our parents' lives been different, would we still be our familiar selves? Impossible questions. Yet they are there. They have engaged the human mind for centuries, and they all point to a mysterious beginning, our own beginning. Whatever that starting moment may have been, we know it is our greatest milestone, because that is where life was created.

When we think of the time of conception, when sperm and egg came together, we feel awe. In that tiny and obscure happening, so infinitesimal and hidden it cannot be seen, so gentle it can hardly be felt, something occurs which bears the dignity and the grandeur of a cosmic event: the birth of human destiny.

Overwhelmingly powerful factors conspire to structure and condition that momentous event, both before and after: the entire course of human evolution and history; the genes, health, mindset, and chemistry of the parents; after birth, again, the family, the immediate group, and this delirious society, with its television, nuclear weapons, high-speed performance, and technological wonders.

But think of that moment when the sperm is incorporated in the egg. That instant transcends the flowing of time, and it is perhaps the only event in our lives when we are totally natural and spontaneous. That instant is also the moment of triumph, when the sperm, after having travelled immense distances, having dodged and overcome obstacles, won the competition with five hundred million other sperms, defied all sorts of traps and perils, finally arrives at the longed-for destination. In some kind of unknowable alchemy a miraculous quantum leap occurs. From a predictable biological happening springs the beginning of a human life, an individual who is capable of loving and hating, of thinking and dreaming, of making wars and composing symphonies. This is the moment of beginning. And all beginnings carry in themselves something hopeful and happy. Beginnings should always be accompanied by enthusiasm, and good wishes, and a loving care, and faith, and thoughts that all is well and all shall be well.

Yet consider what most often happens instead. The most basic and sacred moment of an individual's life is surrounded by the most hurtful of all human attitudes: indifference. This inattention does not occur out of any ill will. The actual time of conception, which usually takes place five or six hours after intercourse, is relegated to indifference and unconsciousness, treated as any routine bodily process, such as digestion, for example. A miracle happens, but nobody is there to witness it: we become too busy with the business of life, too tired and sleeping, or just not confident enough to think one is able to experience such a subtle and minute process. A miracle happens, but nobody is there to watch, to love, to care.

Let us talk a moment, before we go on to happier thoughts, about indifference and its deadly influence on our daily relationships. Just think of the indifference of the busy shopper intent in selecting the best item, unaware of the child in need of a smile; think of our indifference for the ill and the hungry in near and distant countries; or, even more absurd, think of the mutual indifference of people living together, supposedly loving each other, yet unwilling or unable to listen with the heart to the other's dreams and hopes, small victories and tragedies. Indifference is often a convenient cover for the horror and the anger we do not know how to express or deal with. Indifference is deadly because it kills all that is most tender and vulnerable within ourselves and others, which could flower into wonderful relationships and achievements.

We can think of hell as a place of hate, red, aglow with fire, full of trembling and despair. But we may also think of it as a grey region of indifference, where love cannot be expressed because nobody cares and, if it is expressed, goes unnoticed. This hell is a place where nobody pays attention and therefore no fun, no joy exist; where anything precious and original is wasted because it is not heeded; and where, because nobody is generous enough to give of himself, all is clothed with the tired despair of anonymity and nothingness.

Fortunately, the remedy for this hell is available at any moment: it is awareness. Like love and beauty, awareness is a superior moral value. When it is applied to any event in life, chances are that new meaning will dawn. Because of awareness, we are present and able to respond. Instead of forgetting, we remember. Rather than becoming crystallized, we gain in flexibility. The walls of prejudice and fantasy crumble down. We become more receptive and therefore able to enjoy, to relate, and when necessary, to confront pain.

Awareness

For a few moments at a time during the day, be aware. Anything and anybody you meet with can become the subject of your attention:

—what you see, touch, hear, smell, taste;
—feelings, images, thoughts;
—those around you, their moods and expres-
sions.

Don't try to concentrate strenuously on any one
subject or to include everything at once. Try, for
instance, experiencing the taste of an apple, or
your own breathing, or the noise of cars in the
street. Just a few moments of awareness in a day
are a victory.

No subject is better than any other, therefore don't
worry about choice. Be aware of the beautiful
and the ugly, the pleasant and the unpleasant
alike. Do so, if possible, without judging, compar-
ing or adding anything of your own. You will
then be awake and alive. As the great painter
Raphael said when he was asked the secret of his
art, "You will not treat anything as unworthy of
attention."

Also, you will realize how much easier it is to let
yourself be lulled to sleep again by the familiar
routine of everyday thinking. So, if you catch
yourself unaware, bravo! One moment of aware-
ness is worth a hundred centuries of unawareness.

Why do we speak of awareness? Because the gift of
awareness can be applied to conception too. Conscious conception means approaching the moment of life's beginning with all
the attention it deserves. The mother, by remaining in touch
with the psychophysical clues following intercourse, may
become aware of the actual moment when conception takes
place. Several mothers who actually were aware of that moment

have reported that their relationship with that child after it was born was deeper and more open than with their other children.

Awareness can reach much further than the actual moment of conception. It can touch the parents' whole life situation: after making the decision to have a child, the two parents can move towards their highest spiritual, psychological and physical state. Conception means starting an epic adventure that will carry a human being through innumerable worlds, deeds, and possibilities. Then, why not give it a great start? Volumes upon volumes have been written about the process of becoming what we may be. Here we will just enumerate some of the main aspects:

- –a clean nourishing diet: eating whole, fresh food; eliminating those substances which are especially harmful to unborn babies;

- –physical exercise: running, swimming, dancing, yoga, or any other form of bodywork, best if outdoors and in nature;

- –spiritual growth: meditating, contemplating beauty. The cultivation of altruistic love can open us to values immensely greater than our day-to-day self;

- –relationship with partner: The child you are going to create is the result of your relationship. But what is the state of your relationship?

Just think—everything in the universe influences everything else. The fresh fruits and vegetables you ate yesterday; the air you breathe in the forest; the movement in walking or running, vitalizing each cell of your body; a mind alert and full of interests; a state of joy and openness; an honest, warm relationship with your partner. All these elements participate in setting the spiritual, psychological, and chemical environment for the moment of conception, and therefore the life of a human being, his future actions and relationships with you and others. Of course, the scenario could be much different. The psycho-physical environment of conception may be tainted by harmful substances, stale air, and other forms of chronic poisoning; by a mind asleep with no inspiration; and by a relationship with one's partner made of harsh words or ominous silences. Which alternative do you prefer for yourself? And which alternative will you choose for your child?

Preparing for the moment of conception offers you the opportunity for a renewal of your perspective and existence. Rather than being a random moment, lost in the events of ordinary life, conception can turn into the culmination of in-depth work on yourself and your relationships; it can become an illuminating beacon for you now. And what a splendid support for your child's wholeness when you will recount to him with the smallest details the Great Story of your preparation for him: running, singing, praying . . . months or years before he came into the world! The following is a meditation on your relationship with your partner.

You and Your Partner

The atmosphere between you and your partner is going to be the atmosphere in which a human being will be conceived, unfold during pregnancy, be born, and grow. It is the basic environment for a human being in his most vulnerable time. The emotions floating between the two of you, spoken and unspoken, will influence how he or she will be and relate to others. (Please remember that even when the father is absent, a relationship with him still exists.) One of the most favorable times to look at this relationship is now, when it is still possible to change your decision to have a child. Anything you can do towards a better atmosphere, a deeper and renewed closeness, a truer appreciation, and a mutual satisfaction of each other's needs is best started at this time.

You can follow this meditation together with your partner. However, if he or she is not interested or available, you can also work by yourself.

Take some time in becoming aware of the atmosphere between you and your partner: Is it clear? Is it cloudy?

Are there unfinished issues between the two of you, resentments that have not been expressed, questions to be asked, feelings not shared?

Think about your needs. Are there any needs you are expecting your partner to fulfill which he or she doesn't fulfill?

Now close your eyes, and allow yourself to sense the deeper atmosphere in this relationship. Underlying the ever-changing problems and joys on the surface of this relationship, is its unique pattern. Take some time just sensing it.

Now let an image emerge that represents your relationship with your partner. Don't choose it, just let it emerge spontaneously. It can be an image of absolutely anything in the world, real or imaginary, big or small, animate or inanimate, artificial or natural.

Now spend some time with this image. Let it convey its message to you. Allow it to become something else if it wants to.

Open your eyes, share your image with your partner, and discuss its possible meanings with her or him.

Very little is known about conscious conception and the surrounding factors by which it is influenced. All that can be offered is a mixture of fact and hypothesis. To begin with—and this is fact—sperm and egg, and then the fertilized egg, are sensitive to the states of mind and health of mother and father at the moment of conception. These states are at all moments translated into biochemical messages. The physical medium in which conception occurs is generated by man and woman during intercourse and is determined by their psychological and physical state. The hypothesis is that the way in which conception happens—its tempo, ease, and nature—may leave a trace on the entity that comes into being.

In other words, psychological states sometimes affect physical processes subtly and lastingly; and consciousness, feelings, and memory are not the exclusive characteristics of fully developed human beings, but can also be found in the primitive form at the cellular level.

Traces of the memory of one's own conception may, then, lie deeply in our very substance. Dutch psychiatrist Lietaert Peerbolte has discovered, in working with his clients and their dreams, that there are still clear traces within us of that original moment. Dreams are such stuff as we are made of, so there may be something in the daring conjectures he puts forth. Dreams of leaving a whole of some sort, he says, such as a big group of people may symbolize the detachment of the ovum from the ovary. Dreams of moving through a long tunnel or a dark passageway to a place of rest, such as a bed, a chapel or a field full of flowers, may represent the movement of the egg through the oviduct and its arrival, once fertilized, at the uterus. Dreams of airplanes or spaceships full of men in an interplanetary journey may symbolize the travelling sperms from the ovum's point of view. Dreams of collision, of explosion and light may be conception itself.

Likewise, another psychiatrist, Dr. Stan Grof, has found through the visionary imagery evoked in psycholitic therapy that the memories of preconceptual and prenatal events may be as precise as they are clear and colorful. In this approach, imagery is so vivid and detailed that in many cases it is not just the result of the person's imagination, but rather the faithful representation, either symbolic or literal, of actual events in the remote past of the individual or the race.

Similar research could be quoted, showing that the very beginning of our beings still lives within. If this idea seems unlikely, please remember the cave man was not aware of language or mathematical concepts; Napoleon's ideas about outer space or the atomic world would appear naive to any school-child today; and an English eighteenth-century factory worker would find it impossible to believe in the existence of electro-magnetic waves creating colors and shapes on television screens. As saints, scientists, and poets remind us, we are just specks surrounded by unknown realities—our intelligence may not be fully developed, our ethical capacities yet primitive, our perception of beauty still dormant, our senses too dull, our knowledge too limited to comprehend our boundless universe. Rather than arrogantly shrugging off the existence of unknown wonders within and without, let them be inspirations and incentives:

> *Ah! But a man's reach should exceed his grasp*
> *or what's a heaven for.*
> *—Robert Browning*

The Moment of Conception

The following meditation originated from the reports of many people who have recalled the experience of their own conceptions.

As long as you approach the following with an open state of mind, it doesn't matter whether it is memory or imagination or both that are guiding you. Most of all, do not try to prove or disprove anything. The purpose of the meditation is to bring attention to your own conception.

Indeed, what follows is an open guide to your own as well as your future child's conception. As in a musical piece in which the main theme cyclically returns, life constantly repeats itself, each occurrence resonating with the previous ones, yet carrying ever surprising variation. For this reason you are asked to get acquainted with your own conception—in it you may find the source of your original being. Yet we will not stop here. Life dances on. Another identity, completely different, comes now into being: your child.

Precision is not the point in this meditation. On the contrary, give free rein to fantasy and let any feeling and symbolic image emerge. Maybe it is impossible to distinguish reality from fiction. However that may be, this could be the right opportunity for freeing ancient emotional blocks and for reaching back into the very beginning of you.

Lie down, breathe deeply, and for a while let go of the present. Do this for at least five minutes.

Smoothly, gently, you are going back to your own conception, to the hours before sperm penetrates egg. Imagine and feel the time before your conception. How do you experience this state?

A man and a woman have made love. Five hundred million sperm cells are now racing toward their destination, while the egg is waiting for that piercing touch which will begin the miracle of individuation.

The racing legions of sperms are surging, swirling, dashing forward. Like salmon, they must swim upstream against the fluid currents of the oviduct in order to reach the egg. One out of five hundred million will avoid or surmount all the obstacles encountered on its dramatic voyage—a journey proportionally larger and more dangerous than a trip to the moon for a human being. Only one of them will eventually join with the egg. Others will give up the race, while some ease the way for those who have greater mobility and a more compelling impulse toward immortality. Soon the competition will become keener, more desperate. This is a serious race, where only the winner will survive.

You feel both the tranquil and the dynamic waiting of the egg and the compelling race, the fundamental need of the sperm.

Now your own conception takes place. As the egg and the sperm unite, imagine and feel the release of energy, the explosion of light that takes place.

It may be like an explosion of illuminated energy to match the most effulgent sunburst you have ever witnessed. It may be like landing on a faraway planet, or coming home again, or soaring high in the air, or melting with the ocean. It may be a peaceful passivity moving into intense activity. Let your fantasy take whatever shape it wants.

Take time to absorb this experience. Silently and quietly, with your own rhythm, come back to the present. Don't move, and keep your eyes closed. You have explored your own most distant past. After experiencing your own conception, you are now invited to imagine the conception of your future child. Remaining in the same state, without interruptions of any kind, you shift your consciousness from the past toward the future, and envision the conception of your child.

Again visualize vividly the sperm. It is moving quickly, it is pushing forward amidst a crowd of innumerable other sperms. They are doomed to extinction; it alone will win. Imagine this immense, fantastic, new journey; feel the stamina, the strength it takes to fight against all odds; experience in yourself, too, its passionate desire for life, its quest for immortality; imagine this cosmic trip to a faraway, mysterious planet. This is another chance for life, through you, to move on. Together with living energy, the sperm also carries immense amounts of information. Within its DNA coils are enclosed the timeless archives of life, laboratories bursting with activity, precise blueprints and directions for future development.

Now look at the center of the cyclone: the egg. You can perceive its perfect state of receptivity, its peaceful stillness, teeming with infinite possibilities, with prodigious amounts of information. Like the fabled Sleeping Beauty whose unmanifested energies invited the princely touch which would awaken her to consciousness and love, the egg is waiting for the approach of the sperm, which will begin the miracle of individuation.

Now you envision the environment in which the meeting of sperm and egg will take place. What emotional atmosphere would you like it to be? The explosive joy of life, perhaps, or overwhelming tenderness, a peace no words can describe, or the health of life in its most vibrant state. Whatever your preference, like a painter or a composer, you can now create it. You can also imagine its color, consistency, transparency, its smells and sounds.

Finally, the sperm reaches the egg. In that moment a whole universe comes into being. All is contained in it: the initial, cosmic Big Bang, galaxies and stars, the unfolding of the solar system, the dawn of life on our planet, billions of years of evolution. In it, as momentous remnants, live the histories of entire civilizations and their creations. In that coming together pulsates the fate of humankind with its wondrous potential. The conception of your child is taking place now.

Slowly and gradually come back to everyday consciousness.

It is very beautiful to feel the duality, the differentiation of egg and sperm, and then their explosive "becoming one."

This relinquishing of a separate identity and the ensuing fusion into one whole is much more than a purely physiological event: it is a release and an emergence into a more vast consciousness. In numerous instances people have experienced it as a triumphantly divine YES, as a "bliss beyond bliss, all other joys transcending."

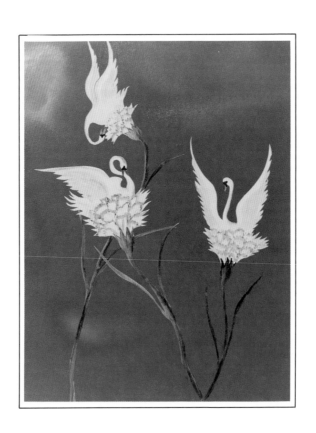

4 Reverence For Life

Goodness is the saving or supporting of life, the enabling of whatever life I can influence to attain its highest development.

–A. Schweitzer

A flower blossom conceals an extraordinary vitality, tireless activity under a seemingly tranquil exterior. Soon the treasure will spring forth and reveal itself in a wonderful show of color and form. But that unfolding, though purposeful and astonishingly precise, is delicate: too much sun, too much rain, and the flower dies.

The full blueprint of a giant oak is hidden in an acorn—an oak which will stand in storm and sunshine, house a multitude of creatures, generate a whole forest. Think of the tremendous energy the oak contains, the delicacy and minuteness of its patterns, the accurate determination of its plans. Yet the acorn is so small, someone could step on it and crush it easily, or inadvertently kick it into a nearby ditch and turn it into nothing. Or imagine a cocoon, so anonymous and so vulnerable, dangling up there from a branch; yet it is a living miracle factory, preparing its astounding legerdemain, from worm to butterfly that will open its wings and wander in space.

The story of the embryo is similar, but even more prodigious. So delicate and concealed, it goes through the fastest, grandest metamorphosis known on the planet. Medical students learning embryology are often awed by the series of transformations an embryo goes through. Each step is a new invention, a quantum leap, completely unpredictable, the ever new production of a most imaginative Mind.

To start understanding this process, you must shift perspective and identify with the point of view of the fetus. You, the fetus, are engaged in the most unbelievable of all journeys. In a few months you are to undergo millions of years of evolution, swiftly summing up all of our history, from amoeba through reptile to apelike to human. Although your development is already set by the ancestral intelligence of the race, you have never been through this process yourself, a process not even a Leonardo or a Shakespeare could ever dream of inventing. You are the future of this planet. The gravest responsibilities, the most dramatic dilemmas, the most tantalizing adventures are awaiting you. Without fear of overstatement you can be called sacred.

And what happens all around you? As it has been conclusively proven, you can hear what goes on outside the womb. But what do you hear? Perhaps harsh or frightening noises or painful fights. Like a dolphin, you live in a vibrational medium. Sounds reach you, distant and dreamlike, yet very real.

As a necessary fuel for your tremendous journey, nourishment comes to you unchosen: it may be healthful or a kind of poison—caffeine, nicotine, or alcohol.

You need a quiet and serene environment, but what do you get? Maybe the emotional medium you are floating in is laden with hostility, despair, and anxiety.

The consequences of anything that happens to you, the fetus, are long-lasting. Pregnancy is both a fragile and a decisive process: fragile, because the slightest disturbance may cause irreparable harm; decisive, because the prenatal environment shapes your future life. Now your body is being created, now it is decided whether you will begin life healthy or unhealthy, weak or strong. Also, the deepest dispositions of your psyche, your most ingrained existential attitudes, may well originate during this period.

In this process, event becomes structure. An event—an act of kindness, a fight, an accident, your mother's anxiety—is experienced by you as a terrific cataclysm or as a pleasant release. And this event becomes structure—in the formation of body tissue or as a deeply ingrained character trait.

During this time, mother is the universe for you. She is all there is, she is your sun, moon and stars, she is trees and rivers and birds. And she is there all the time, inexorably present. "Universe" is to us adults the place we live in, the people we meet every day, the sounds we hear, the food we eat, the bed we sleep in. Even in the most restricted life there is some kind of escape. But you, the fetus, have no choice: those few cubic inches of universe you live in, that is your All, the beginning of your character, your philosophy, your attitude toward the world. Moreover, a relatively stable condition, rhythmic heart-beat, no distractions or alternatives, semi-darkness, complete vulnerability, no possibility of objection, make this the perfect situation for suggestion and imprinting. So defenseless and at the same time so busy with miraculous unfolding, are you trapped in the tightest and most pitiless clutch? Or, as in a nightmare, bumped and shoved this way and that? Or frozen in the misery of rejection? Or floating in the heaven of tenderness?

The first relationship you experience is the closest one. And this medium is where the blueprint for your future is set: truly, *health and disease, love and hate, war and peace, start in the womb.*

The great Swiss psychologist, C.G. Jung, claimed that our prenatal relationship with our mothers lives on in our unconscious, imagery and dreams in two main ways: positive—for example a fountain that nourishes and regenerates, food and drink of the most wonderful kind, the fertile earth, or the ocean; or negative—a cold tomb where you are inescapably trapped, a swamp or a sticky marsh, sinister vegetation that encloses you, a web you cannot escape where you fall prey to a monstrous spider.

The difference starts in the womb. Now more than any other time is the period for you, the mother, to be kind to yourself and to your child. This kindness, this reverence for all that lives, is likely to open you to a beautiful awareness, to help you feel part of a whole incomparably greater than yourself. Albert Schweitzer wrote:

> You walk outside and it is snowing. You carelessly shake the snow from your sleeves. It attracts your attention: a lacy snowflake glistens in your hand. You can't help looking at it. See how it sparkles in a wonderfully intricate pattern. Then it quivers, and lies dead in your hand. It is no more. The snowflake which fluttered down from infinite space upon your hand, where it sparkled and quivered and died—that is yourself. Wherever you see life—that is yourself!

Even more important, your kindness is going to have long-lasting consequences; it will become part of a body and may reverberate for years in the child and, therefore, in other persons' lives. Unfortunately, as we all know, the world is full of people who make it their special pastime to be unkind to themselves. Don't be too quick to rule yourself out: the forms of self-destructiveness are infinite. We may just forget to take enough care of ourselves, or not feel worthy enough to deserve pleasure, rest, and self-nourishment; we may not be able to be open and receive what people who love us are offering; as in the slowest of suicides, we may routinely introduce toxic substances into our bodies; in order to avoid loneliness, we may take all sorts of indignity and injustice from the people we meet; we may torture ourselves with guilt; we may be too shy to risk expressing what we know is right and beautiful.

Mother, this is the time to be kind to yourself—by eating nourishing food; by caring for yourself and taking time to rest; by offering yourself any delight, large or small, you can think of and afford. It is as if your womb were a microcosm: love affairs and warfare, sickness and the full bloom of vigor, gentleness and violence, everything takes on a more dramatic prominence and carries a greater weight for the future development of your child.

Though not an illness, as it was sometimes regarded in the past, pregnancy can be a troubled time. Many new and perhaps unpleasant sensations arise. The strangest feelings may emerge, ups and downs may be the rule. Besides, life goes on with all its unpredictable quirks. Perhaps you are a working woman. You have very little time and even earning a little money is a struggle. Perhaps this pregnancy makes you particularly uncomfortable, and your body is not quite fit for it. Maybe the man who created this child with you does not even know about it, has left you, or is far away just when you most need comfort and assurance. Maybe this pregnancy meets with disapproval and skepticism from those who are close to you. And perhaps you are alone.

Yet you are having this baby, and whoever you are and whatever your difficulties may be, you are hosting the most wondrous of all developments. Thus, if you can take even five minutes a day, to think good thoughts, listen to your favorite music, or nourish yourself in any way you want, your kindness will be multiplied a thousandfold and become an organic part of a person's being for years to come. Five minutes of care is worth years of well-being. What's more, you can talk to the embryo, sending it warm, reassuring messages, even verbal ones. And what would *he* tell *you*?

Perhaps, "My heart beats today for the first time," or "I am becoming a female or a male, I have lungs now, I can move my legs and arms, I can start seeing and hearing, I have developed a million new brain cells today." Or, in a cry of joyous emergency, "I am ready! I am ready to be born!"

So there can be a dialogue going on between you and your embryo or fetus. In fact, a dialogue is going on all the time, if by that we mean an exchange of messages, in the form of feelings and sensations. And all this, of course, is translated into a chemical dance of the most fateful kind, a dance which will decide whether this being will begin life confident or insecure, healthy or unhealthy, loving or unloving.

Dialogue with the Unborn

In the imagery that follows, you, the future mother or the future father, will be led to meet your unborn child and dialogue with it. Should you decide to do this imagery together, please remember not to give each other ideas or suggestions. During this meditation silence is of the essence. It will be a very special dialogue, because the unborn, though human, does not yet belong to your world and knows nothing of your reality. It will be like a dialogue with a being from another planet, living in totally different conditions than your own. And yet this being is infinitely close to you, it is a part of you. For the time being its destiny is your destiny, its body is your own body; therefore a subtle communication can begin to happen. The only way to make this dialogue fruitful is for you to make yourself as receptive as he or she is, and to listen deeply, consciously, openly.

Close your eyes, relax for a few moments, and pay attention to your breathing. Don't force it, but, feeling you have all the time in the world, let it get deeper and slower.

As you pay attention to your breath, you become more attentive. For the time being, leave behind your daily cares, your opinions, your habits, even your needs. Let your breathing take care of itself. You are silent consciousness.

As a silent presence, you find that your awareness is becoming vaster, deeper. You are open to what is, and receptive in all directions. There is nothing verbal about this awareness. Naked awareness, stripped of all concepts, is particularly sensitive to even the subtlest feelings, sensations, and intimations.

As pure consciousness you can be anywhere: in the depths of the ocean or on top of a mountain peak, on a deserted beach or in a forest, inside a leaf or on a rainbow, in the center of the earth or on a star.

Of all the possible places within your reach, you choose the dark, enchanted dwelling of the unborn where you will meet the child of your dreams. You will journey to the mysterious abode where human life begins.

You travel now through layers of flesh and placenta, through the wondrous geometry of cells, through pulsating blood, in veins and dark spaces, through the living factory of inner organs, through amazing landscapes, towards that deep place where life is created.

You reach the place where the unborn is living. A tiny heart is beating; a form is slowly undulating in this liquid medium, suspended in space. The eyes do not yet see the forms we are so familiar with: they are still open to infinity. You have an impression of something powerful and sublime at work here; with precise pace, with timeless knowing, all is developing. You are there, you are conscious. You sense the presence of a being. It is your child.

Take some time, now, to establish a contact with this presence. For the time being—in this place, so dark yet teeming with life's energy—you just receive. You are totally attentive now, open to any message that may come to you.

You listen. The presence of the unborn is itself a communication. You sense its mood, its state of being. As you set your assumptions aside, messages reach you with surprising clarity.

Now the unborn is communicating with you in a more active way.

Listen! It tells you where it comes from.

Listen! It tells you about its life now.

Listen! It tells you its wishes, its needs.

Listen! It tells you about its possibilities and the future. (As you hear about them, please don't let your own wishes and projects come in the way.)

Now it's your turn to communicate. You can express whatever you feel is of value to this being.

You may want to project towards it a wordless flow of warmth and embracing tenderness, the joy of knowing that it exists. You can transmit to it images of all that is most beautiful in this world your child will be coming into. You may communicate with it with music—peaceful lullabies, happy songs. You could even talk to it with words, soothing and reassuring words. The way or ways of communication are up to you.

You can continue this dialogue as long as you like, and repeat it again and again. You will thus have created the deepest relationship: the prenatal bond.

This is cosmic imagery, reaching into the most mysterious aspects of our existence. Yet imagination and feeling, though the central guiding factor for you at this time, can be usefully complemented by the positive support of fact. In this realm, facts may confirm what, deep down, you already know. And, remember, at this time even a small advantage becomes a lifelong benefit. These are realities you may find useful to know:

* Bad food for the mother is poison for the fetus.

The theory used to be that even if the mother were malnourished, the fetus managed in some miraculous way to draw from her the nutrients in the right proportions and needed quantities. Not so. Food that is wholesome, varied, fresh, and nourishing has an enormous value for the baby, especially its brain cells.

* The fetus lives in a world full of sounds and lights.

First of all, the unborn hears the inner sounds of mother's body: the pulsations of the heart and the rumbling of the intestines, for instance. It will also react to external sounds—music, for example—in rather differentiated ways: by preferring, perhaps, Mozart to Wagner, or classical to rock. As some experiments have shown, fetuses have their own distinctive taste and are quite capable of liking one kind of music while reacting against another (this fact can be detected by measuring the fetus's heart rate).

Music has also been employed to imprint a fetus. In one study, the same rhythmical piece was played several times so the unborn could hear it; later, when the same music was played to the newborn, it had a soothing and beneficial influence, as if showing a reassuring continuity between the womb and the real world out there—very useful in case of stressful birth circumstances and environment. Also, positive reactions to that same piece continued for months after birth.

Then, of course, there are the ordinary sounds of everyday living, especially voices in conversation. Through them, events of the mother's life write their story deeply in the fetus's dawning psyche. Finally, a fetus reacts to light stimuli. A sharp light startles it. A soft one causes the fetus to gently turn toward it.

* The fetus is active.

In his article "The Fetus as Personality," Albert W. Liley tells us:

> Far from being an inert passenger in a pregnant mother, the fetus is very much in command of the pregnancy. It is the fetus who guarantees . . . the endocrine success of the pregnancy and induces all manner of changes in maternal physiology to make her a suitable host . . . it is the fetus who decides which way he will lie in pregnancy and which way he will present labor. Even in labor the fetus is not entirely passive—neither the toothpaste in the tube nor the cork in the champagne bottle as required by the old hydraulic theories of the mechanics of labor.

* The fetus is strongly affected by the emotional life of the mother.

The amount of data on this subject is overwhelming and often offers horrendous instances. The essence, however, is evident: "Emotional difficulties in the mother," says Ashley Montagu, "are biochemical, electrical, and reverberative." Thus a subjective event can affect the formation of even the most solid tissue, such as the bones. "This much is clear: the emotions of a pregnant woman do have an effect on her child before he is born, in the form of chemicals and hormones sent to him from her circulation through the placenta to his blood stream."

* The father's quality of presence is important.

Father, you are pregnant too. Your relationship with the woman in your life at this time is second in importance only to her relationship with the fetus. Obviously enough, the way you treat her has a direct influence on her own feelings of self-worth and well-being, and therefore an indirect but most powerful influence on the child. And let us not forget your voice. Possibly, with the exception of mother's, yours is the voice the fetus will hear most, and it will contribute to its vibratory universe: rage or tenderness, joy or cruelty in your words will reach it deep down in its hidden world. You may feel excluded and foreign at first to what is going on, yet you need not, for the support you are willing to offer can be more important than ever. To put it bluntly, how are you going to contribute? Just by donating your sperm, or also your soul? This may be the time for you to decide whether you want to be an absent or a present father.

Now, after fact comes speculation. We have seen how vulnerable the fetus is to the feelings of mother. Yet the only proof may be empathy or imagination. Perhaps the human being will never again be so moldable and open to impression as during the prenatal existence. You, the mother, may choose on the basis of this hypothesis, not to expose this impressionable organism to the random effects of the inner and outer events of your everyday life. Instead you may wish to choose carefully your environments. You can surround yourself with what you feel is most beautiful in works of art, especially music. The esthetic experience can be as simple as a few color reproductions and music on the radio. Or, at the very least, you may be wary of opening yourself up to the confusion and the ugliness of much of the mass media material. You could also expose yourself to the profound, pervading influence of nature—forests, mountains, sky.

You could use some of your time during pregnancy for learning the art of meditation to explore yourself and intentionally induce positive states of mind, as far as the emotional ups and downs, so common during this period, will allow you. One way of doing so is by cultivating qualities such as peace, joy, strength, love, beauty, and so on. During the nine months of pregnancy, you may meditate on a different quality each month.

Of course, concentrating on a Botticelli painting won't make your child look like a Venus. The genetic program is going to take its own inevitable course. The unborn child will develop whether the environment is one of rage, pain, and ugliness, or one of beauty and joy. Yet, knowing how deeply and lastingly such aspects can affect a human being, it seems natural that they affect a human being in the making.

Suppose, however, that the idea of a close psychological relationship between mother and fetus is a myth. In this case, the pregnant mother can still benefit by following these suggestions. First, she will have a pleasant time and perhaps learn something of value. She may develop a greater sense of self-esteem and self-respect—attitudes so needed by her now and always.

Secondly, while the day-to-day trials of the pregnancy induce a bond between the mother and the fetus, an even more exquisite aspect of that relationship is offered by what we are suggesting, for the mother will later tend to create naturally an association between the beauty with which she comes in contact and her future child. Such prolonged effort can only enhance her enjoyment of her child. This is yet another benefit of the "yoga of pregnancy."

To conclude, pregnancy is the most intimate relationship between the creator and the created. For two human beings united and nurtured by love and intelligence, life is not just a struggle for survival, nor is it necessarily easy and comfortable—but it has vibrancy, meaning, and, at times, a touch of nobility.

Envisioning a Quality of Life

The following is a meditation for pregnant mothers (fathers can participate as well):

Choose a quality with which to pervade yourself and your unborn child: joy, beauty, strength, health, serenity . . .

Close your eyes, and let a time emerge during which you have experienced that quality. Do more than just remember, rather allow yourself to relive this situation. Open the door to all feelings and sensations connected with it.

Allow an image to spontaneously emerge which represents the quality you have chosen. It may be absolutely any image: an object or an animal, a galaxy or a flower, an abstract shape or a person. Visualize this picture as clearly as you can.

Now become *that image. Experience what it feels to actually be it.*

For a while, think *about the chosen quality. Think about its value, its beauty and significance. What would your life be like if you had more of that quality? And what could your child's life become if he, or she, were a full expression of it? Imagine these possibilities even in concrete ways, without becoming particularly attached to any of them.*

Before ending this meditation, spend some time in sensing the quality in your body, vibrating in each cell, gradually but powerfully pervading you and your child.

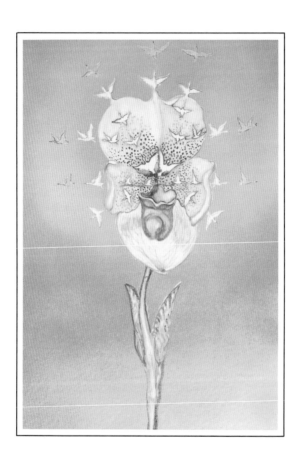

5 O Nobly Born

*All appeared new, and strange at first,
inexpressibly rare and delightful and beautiful. I was
a little stranger, which at my entrance into the world
was saluted and surrounded with innumberable joys
. . . All things were spotless and pure and glorious:
yea, and infinitely mine, and joyful and precious. I
knew not that there were any sins, or complaints or
laws. I dreamed not of poverties, contentions or vices.
All tears and quarrels were hidden from mine eyes.
Everything was at rest, free and immortal. I knew
nothing of sickness or death or rents or exaction,
either for tribute or bread. In the absence of these I
was entertained like an Angel with the works of God
in their splendour and glory, I saw all in the peace of
Eden; Heaven and Earth did sing my Creator's
praises, and could not make more melody to Adam
than to me. All Time was Eternity, and a perpetual
Sabbath. Is it not strange that an infant should be
heir to the whole World, and see those mysteries
which the books of the learned never unfold?*

—Thomas Traherne

It was very early morning, still dark, and raining hard. Dr. Grantly Dick-Read, then a young gynecologist at the beginning of his career, had been called to assist a childbirth. Laboriously finding his way through a maze of alleys in Whitechapel, London's poorest slum, the doctor finally arrived, stumbled up a dark staircase, and found the woman. She was lying in the midst of a room ten feet square, where rain was pouring in through a broken window. Light came from a candle on top of a beer bottle, and the only assistance was given by a sympathetic neighbor. The woman was covered with sacks and an old shirt. Darkness, poverty, and dirt prevailed everywhere one could lay eyes on. Yet the atmosphere was pervaded by tranquillity and kindness, and childbirth was remarkably easy. Only at one moment did some dissension come up: when Dr. Dick-Read had asked his patient if she wanted chloroform—a standard procedure at the time for anesthesia during childbirth—the woman had strangely refused.

The doctor thus continues his story:

> As I was about to leave some time later, I asked her why it was she would not use the mask. She did not answer at once, but looked from the old woman who had been assisting, to the window through which was bursting the first light of the dawn; then shyly she turned to me and said: "It didn't hurt. It wasn't meant to, was it doctor?"
>
> For weeks and months afterwards, as I sat with women in labor, women who appeared to be in terror and agony of childbirth, that sentence came running back in my ears—"It wasn't meant to, was it, doctor?"—until finally, even through my orthodox and conservative mind, I began to see light. I began to realize there was no law in nature and no design that could justify the pain of childbirth.

Perhaps, as Dr. Dick-Read did seventy years ago, it is time to take a new look at birth. As are all fundamental issues, birth is covered by layer after layer of ideas and images that keep us from really seeing what it is. Ideas and images generate emotions and muscular reactions, chemical and—yes—structural changes. This pattern becomes deeply ingrained and is transmitted to us at that very vulnerable moment of our lives—birth. Thus, as we grow up, it remains imprinted in the depth of our bodymind.

But suppose we had the option of thinking about birth anew. Free from ancient conditionings, and mindful of the fundamental power of the imagination, how would we want to envision it? Images and sounds immediately come to mind: sounds of the childbearing woman that, mixed as they may be with groans and toil, are also expressing joy and pleasure, the pleasure of an organism accomplishing what it was designed for, without pressures or interferences; the joy of having brought to light a living creature; images of a baby like a little Buddha, her face peaceful, her eyes immensely aware, pervaded by innocence and the infinity from which she comes; images of a family where the father, too, can be present and participating. Yes, all this is possible and is happening more and more.

By putting aside the preconceived negative images which surround birth, it is possible in most cases to eliminate unnecessary suffering and meet in a serene way the experience of labor. The French doctor Michel Odent, who limits medical intervention as much as possible, strongly believes we should interfere with the natural process only in emergencies. His guiding principle which is perhaps the clearest of all is that birth should be surrounded by the same kind of beautiful and tender environment as lovemaking. A birth taking place under Odent's direction is a good example:

> She, the mother, knows exactly what to do and needs no instructions, because she is so completely in tune with her own body and with the energy that is rushing through it in great waves of desire to push the baby down. The midwife waits, hands resting, occasionally whispering, "Good . . . good." Suddenly the woman lets out a long, low moan and

there is the top of the baby's head, already born. The midwife still waits. And with the next contraction the woman gives a cry that seems one of astonishment and jubilation and pain and triumph—perhaps also of ecstasy—mingled in one great shout. The baby's head slips through, and then the whole body tumbles out onto the cloth that is spread to receive it. Immediately the mother looks down, scoops up her baby, and lifts it to her breast: "I can't believe it! It's incredible! Don't cry, little one! My baby! My baby! Fantastic! Incredible!" she exclaims over and over again, eyes shining and wet with tears, laughing and crying at the same time. She is in her husband's arms and he is kissing her. Nobody intrudes. He kisses the baby's foot, then his wife again. He is crying with the joy and wonder of it, too. This is what birth is like for some women. This is what birth can be.

Unfortunately, it could also be, and often is, something quite different. Influenced by centuries of tradition, by fear, by negative thoughts, and by practices that have estranged us from nature, we picture birth in an entirely different way. The mother is treated as a sick person without control over what is happening to her, and is heavily numbed. When the infant first cries, its very first breath of life coincides with an outraged sound of violated sensitivity. Newborns still bear on their face the traces of terror and pain, as in the most horrified of all surprises—is this what the world is like? Father is estranged and unimportant, pacing and smoking, trying to hide his anxiety and confused feelings, left out of an event that will change all their lives. These negative mental images are transformed into muscular tensions, emotional atmosphere, and chemical environment, and issue a most powerful warning to the newborn: you will make your way through impossible odds, you will ever meet with struggle and tragedy. This message is sculpted deeply in the baby, becoming part of his organism and emotional make-up.

Before you read further, please become aware of your own bodymind. Perhaps your muscles have tensed, your breathing has become shallower, your whole being has contracted. We may have triggered in you some deep, unconscious memory of your own birth and its heavily charged images. We suggest that before you go on, you breathe deeply and slowly a few times. You can let each breath take you closer to that place in yourself which is untouched by all impressions, where the dramas of life have left no trace. There, everything is still possible, no thought is absurd, and you can see everything as if for the first time. There, again, you can reconnect with the happy, serene images of birth. The scenario is once more what it should be: reduced muscle tension, an atmosphere of relaxation, and a welcoming expectation. These surroundings have a deep effect on the newborn. They communicate the most essential message: welcome into a peaceful world, into an atmosphere of joy.

Your Ideal Birth

In this meditation you will not be asked to relive your actual birth, nor to make any comparison with it. Rather, you will create your own birth as you would have liked it to be. The purpose here is to clear up your own feelings about birth and to become aware of it as an opportunity for love, a healthy connection with the universe around us, and a hopeful beginning.

Close your eyes, relax for a while, then let come into your mind a vivid image of the place where you are going to be born. Look at this place, smell its fragrance, and let go of your present body. You are newly born, and you feel whatever is in contact with your tender skin. You are very sensitive, and you feel the vibrations all around you—the vibrations of love and welcome. There is a deep natural peace in this birth, and you feel encircled by all the beings you love and respect. You have the whole creation ready to welcome you. You see your favorite flower, that with its beauty and fragrance tells you, "Welcome, I am happy you are born! Welcome into the world, into the world of flowers."

Now look at the creatures that welcome you. You might choose your favorite animal to help you come into the world—perhaps a dog or a dolphin or a butterfly. You feel this creature and you see it. It too tells you, "Welcome, I am happy you are born! Welcome into the world, into the world of creatures."

Now you see the stars in the cosmos, twinkling everywhere. They too are speaking to you. They are saying, "Welcome, I am happy you are born! Welcome into the world, into the world of stars."

You feel this entrance into a world that respects and welcomes you. You feel love enveloping you. You breathe it, so that it circulates in your bodymind. You feel this joy of entering life, of entering a world where you can do so many beautiful things, where you have the potential of giving love and beauty to yourself and others.

Now think of some of the great people in the history of the world—painters, philosophers, poets. Your favorite ones are there; they all have convened here to welcome you into the world. In their great knowledge there is a great love too. Beauty, intelligence and love, all together are here to welcome you into this birth. You are a miracle, and everyone has come to tell you so. It has taken millions of years of evolution to produce you, noble being with godlike potentialities. And flowers, animals and people are here to remind you, to tell you: you are noble, you are beautiful—you are loved.

And in this birth there is joy. You see smiling faces, smiling flowers, dolphins dancing around you. The whole creation rejoices because you are born!

Let this beauty sink deep into you, and meet with your own beauty. You enter a world where everyone is caring, especially the babies, and you are one of them. It is a world where giving and receiving are just as natural as breathing. You are grateful for this new world. And gratefulness is heaven itself.

True, there are hard realities to be faced in childbirth. From the baby's point of view, this transition—the time before birth and immediately following—is comparable to a cosmic cataclysm. From a condition of unity, being one with mother, the baby enters one of duality. It is the moment when, according to Freud and Rank, anxiety begins. The contact with the unknown totality of the external world is staggering; the newborn's biological rhythms, physical functions—especially breathing—and mode of being undergo a sudden, dramatic change. In fact, for her the whole universe abruptly changes. For these reasons there is much to learn by turning our attention to the baby's point of view. Let's listen, she is speaking to us, the people out there. She is asking something: "Please, let me know that everything is all right. Unlike you, I know nothing, I am innocent and surprised by the world. I am sensitive; therefore don't offend me with loud noises, strong lights, or those hard, cold surfaces. Unlike you, I am not yet used to such intrusions. Please, give me tenderness, closeness, and warmth. I am frightened by having only empty space around me. I need the contact of skin, and where is my mother's heartbeat? I am a stranger in this universe. I just gave up my world, everything is new here. This is my life starting. Be present and awake with me.''

Yes, awake. Everything seems to point in that direction. For months you, the mother, have been carrying this baby. You have felt her weight in your own body, and sensed her kicks and movements. You have wondered what she was like, and yet you have never met her face to face. You could not wait till her birth, but the months, the days, were passing so slowly. You were curious. Now, finally, the culmination has come. Now the rhythm of events has suddenly accelerated. It is the time of birth and your whole being is engaged. As in the best staged of all stories, nature has created this unfolding as if to request total alertness.

This is an exceptional moment. In most of our life's activities, we are given a second chance; perhaps we can rehearse and have ample time to repeat an experience. But the moment of our birth is unique; we are only born once. It is a solemn time. Compared with it, all the rest is prose.

This is the moment of creation. Whether it is the beginning of a galaxy, or a human being, birth is nature at its best. This is the time when all is new and fresh, when life is in its most triumphant state. Birth is the joyous spring of life, gushing from the mystery of an unknown, deep center.

In the midst of a whirlwind of sparkling drops we can imagine a baby. With her entire organism, she impellingly knows her time has come. Her whole being is a vibrant YES that pushes and surges upwards, toward the air and the sun. This baby, marvelously strong and buoyant, is new, yet carries the strength of eons of evolution. She is defenseless, yet exudes the vigor of life. She is coming up from darkness, but is effulgent with light.

No wonder we so easily associate water with birth. The liquid element is the principal primordial source from which we originated, both as individuals in the womb and, in ages past, as the human race.

If the mother's experience at birth is creative, aware, and satisfying, her relationship with the newborn will be immensely happier and more fertile. But if this relationship is marred by unconsciousness and useless pain, this moment of crisis will be left unresolved, and crystallize into chronic difficulties at a later time.

Many approaches have stressed the importance for the woman to consciously and creatively participate in the birth. Sheila Kitzinger states that the woman "no longer hands over her body to doctor and nurses to deal with as they think best. She retains the power of self-direction, of self-control, of choice, of voluntary decision and active cooperation with doctor and nurse." This new attitude toward childbearing is not dependent on technique only—it is basic to one's relationship to life and the universe. It reflects the part one plays in the order of things.

Finally, what about the father and childbirth? What is his role? In the childbirth-with-father approach, pioneer Dr. Robert A. Bradley came to the conclusion that fathers must be part of this joyful event after noticing how much love and gratitude was directed to himself by mothers who had just given birth to their child—while the fathers were waiting elsewhere, anxious, isolated, and excluded from this most meaningful phase of their life together. "As long as the father has been properly trained and is acquainted with the various aspects and phases of labor, he can most profitably participate in the experience. He can provide an invaluable support to his wife, successfully blend with the team in the delivery room, bring an element of joy and humor," and start a bonding relationship with the baby, which will decisively influence their relationship.

Birth Day

The birth of your baby is due soon. You are counting the days now. The following meditation is helpful to generate a beautiful atmosphere for your baby; to help you, the mother, to be more serene and relaxed; and also you, the father, to participate in this memorable event.

Lie down, and, for a long while, as long as it feels comfortable, breathe.

Breathe deeply and slowly. Imagine that all cares, all tensions, all preconceived notions of birth, in fact all thoughts, are leaving you with each exhalation.

Imagine that the air, rather than coming in and out through the nose or mouth, is penetrating you through the whole surface of your body: the entire surface of your skin has become your breathing organ. Take a lot of time to learn to breathe in this new way. Without forcing, let your breathing become deeper and deeper.

As you breathe with your whole body, become aware of the air you breathe. Feel, imagine, that this air is vibrating with vital energy—that it penetrates everywhere in your body: where you are tired, it regenerates you; where you are tense, it relaxes you; where you feel empty, it fills you with light and life.

Now you are going to create the environment in which you want to welcome the baby into the world. Where would you like your child to be born?

—near the ocean, amidst the shells and the splashes and the balmy smell of the sea . . .

—at night, pervaded by silence, under the stars . . .

— under a giant oak, feeling its ancient strength . . .

—during spring, in the midst of a meadow full of flowers of all colors . . .

—in ripe wheat, experiencing the fertility and richness of the earth . . .

—under a gentle rain or a rainbow . . .

—near a waterfall . . .

—on the mountains, surrounded by pure, crisp mountain air . . .

—at dawn or sunset.

These are just a few examples. It is up to you to imagine the environment you prefer. Whatever the setting you have chosen, visualize it as clearly as you can. Imagine actually being there. Breathe, feel the smell, the tactile sensations, hear the sounds and see the colors vividly. As you repeat this exercise, images will become more alive and richer, so do not be discouraged if you do not succeed at first. By visualizing the same setting again, and again, you will make it more and more alive. Whatever your outer environment will be, within the vast space of your mind and through the resources of your imagination, you will actually be creating a living reality in your inner world—and in the inner world of your baby.

Imagine your baby is there with you, newly born. Communicate with your baby with words or songs or through your skin. Talk to him or her about this new world he/she is being born into. Surround your baby with a tender, loving welcome.

As you open your eyes, and slowly, very slowly, come back to everyday consciousness, draw or paint the setting you have chosen for your child to be born in. Remember, perfection and style have no relevance here. You will just express in any way that is easy to you the feelings and the images you have had.

Keep this drawing or painting: it will be part of the Great Story you will tell your child years from now.

In the Tibetan tradition ''O Nobly Born'' is the salutation repeatedly given to a dying person. But why reserve this respect only for the dying? Why not show it to the defenseless newly born who has a whole life to share? The simple thought of a newborn can fill us with wonder and hope. A baby is at the beginning of time, facing countless possibilities. Later events and encounters will set inevitable boundaries. But not yet. We know that the newborn's life will touch thousands of other lives. Will she be the harbinger of warmth and kindliness, or of hostility and despair? Will she treat others in a fair manner, or just take advantage of them—and how will she be treated in return? Holding this baby in our arms, we hold a whole world of possibilities, a microcosm of the future. Unlike us, older and captives of time, she is ready and new. Let us infuse her with our hope and our affection at the start of her great adventure of life. "O Nobly Born!" This is how every new baby should be welcomed. It will be a deep reminder for the rest of her life that she is a beautiful and noble being.

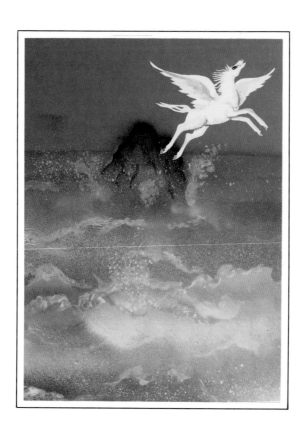

6 *Meeting the World*

What is the little one thinking about?
Very wonderful things no doubt:
Unwritten history!
Unfathomed mystery!
Yet he laughs and cries, and eats and drinks,
And chuckles and crows, and nods and winks,
As if his head were as full of kinks
And curious riddles as any sphinx!

—J.G. Holland

So the baby is born. After all the excitement, the stress, the exultation, he is right there, a new person in your life, a new inhabitant on this planet. Gone are the friends and relatives who came to see the newborn and wish the best; if you had the baby in the hospital, you are now back home. All of the equipment you had prepared with such expectancy in the past weeks—crib, blankets and so on—is ready. This is a great beginning and a true revolution. It is also, however, a continuation. In fact, from the baby's point of view, little has changed. Believe it or not, the great paradox is that, perhaps without realizing it, you are still pregnant.

Usually, the time we call pregnancy is, as we all know, nine months long. At the moment of birth, however, the baby is only half-gestated. He is a fetus still in the process of developing, retaining the vulnerability and the fast-growing pace he had in the uterus. In fact, such are the analogies between the nine months inside the womb and the first months outside that some researchers assure us that the real gestation is actually eighteen months long. They call the two phases utero-gestation and extero-gestation. So the newborn is still in the womb, but now "a womb with a view," as Ashley Montagu put it. And the mother, when she follows nature's course, retains an almost continuous physical contact with the baby, protects him from stimuli which are too strong, and surrounds him with warmth and protection. Thus the unfolding which had started nine months before can continue its course in the best of conditions, while the baby very, very gradually adapts to the external environment. At the end of this period the baby, as a first faint statement of his independence, will be able to crawl.

This being is infinitely delicate. Imagine a budding rose, its tenderest inner folds, its secret treasure preparing to manifest, barely starting to emit its perfume and to show its future beauty, a living project which outer elements could unconsciously, but pitilessly, hurt. Now the prodigious results of the nine months of creation are coming to light. With perfect timing nature, the amazing stage master, abandons all secrecy and shows off her magic in all its delicacy and splendor. And what life and potential, what radiant promises, what hope, are in that blossom—or in that baby! And yet, what a tremendous vulnerability!

Who can imagine a better and more beautiful relationship than the one between mother and newborn? Nature made it so perfect, esthetically, chemically, physiologically. All rhythms and functions are in perfect harmony as long as no artificial interference disturbs them. The gaze between the mother's and baby's eyes, for instance, so intense and direct, seems to say, "We are born to be related. We are relationship." Ah, if only we could for a moment forget all of our reservations and fears and relate with each other with the same unobstructed presence and trust, what would the world be like then? How ridiculous our games and our wars would look! And yet this is what we were born to be.

Now the ritual of breastfeeding has started. The faintest baby's sigh is enough to start milk secretion and nipple erection in the mother. The exchange of skin contact and warmth is precisely what gives most pleasure to both. In this magic intimacy a deep bond is starting, which can continue for the rest of these people's lives. And what a perfect surrender may be seen in these two creatures: all the triviality, the redundancy, the pretense we have painstakingly woven into the fabric of our adulthood is completely absent here. This surrender and innocence remind us of the cleanliness of a waterfall, the stillness of a forest, or the purity of the stars, where everything is exactly what it is: no more, no less.

So the Great Story goes on with continuously new episodes and developments. Think of a later time, when you will describe to your child his first smile and the way his eyes looked at you, perfectly open, living still in another world of infinite space. Or perhaps the subject of your stories will be more practical: the time you went to buy the cradle, uncle's funny reaction when first seeing the newborn, or the story of how both of his parents were turned into sleepy ghosts by this infant who had not yet fully realized the night is made for sleeping. Maybe you will be able to find words to describe the profound stillness of your baby's sleep or how soft his skin felt. Perhaps words will fail you, and you will suddenly start singing the old, favorite lullaby—and you will see in his expression a look of surprised, delighted recognition of the rhythm that rocked him into life.

There is a special charm about this time in your life with your newborn. But this magic should not prevent us from forgetting the decisive quality of this period: your relationship with your baby is at a crossroads. It may be reinforced, so that it will fully bloom and establish itself in a stable manner. But it can also be irreversibly harmed. During the sensitive period immediately after birth, if mother and father maintain a close contact with the newborn, their relationship with him will later be of a much more satisfactory quality. Studies have shown that mothers who were able to be close to their babies right after birth, as compared with those who could only get a few glimpses of him, showed more concern, more tenderness, and more fondling. By the time the children were about five, the early contact group showed a better command of language and a higher intelligence.

In addition, close observation of videotape sequences has revealed that the psychophysical relationship between mother and infants is extraordinarily subtle and has all the best attributes of a dance. As the baby looks at his mother, he moves in ballet-like movements; if the mother falls out of step in this dance by not responding appropriately, the baby keeps trying to get her attention. And if he fails, he then collapses in a state of helplessness, turns his face aside, and remains motionless.

The profound, almost uncanny power of the bonding relationship becomes particularly evident in those rare cases where the mother is mistakenly given the wrong baby. After several days, when the mistake is found, the mother can have her own baby again. However, she has grown so atttached to the "wrong" baby that she does not want to separate from him, and only reluctantly, and after repeated insistence, does she agree to have the mistake corrected and return to the natural baby. Episodes of this kind show that early bonding may create a relationship stronger than genes—an encouraging fact for all those who adopt a baby immediately after birth.

Bonding has another beneficial effect on the baby—it helps him to reorganize his rhythms. As a newborn adapts to the extrauterine environment, he also needs to adjust his biological rhythms such as sleep, for instance, to his new condition. The physical proximity of the mother greatly helps in re-establishing this "biorhythmicity." The role of the mother in this respect has been compared to a magnet's action in lining up iron filings.

Another interesting effect that early contact has on mothers is to increase their tendency to hold the baby to hear their heartbeats, which has a beneficial influence on the child. Apparently, when this happens during the baby's first days of life, his weight increases at a more substantial rate. Also, the newborn is easily soothed the moment he can hear a tape of mother's heartbeat.

Early exposure to the father also significantly helps to form a close tie. This attitude of "engrossment" of the father has been described as "attraction to the infant, perception of the newborn as perfect, extreme elation and increased sense of self-esteem." Babies who have been touched and held by the father during this sensitive period have been shown to cope better with stress nine months later.

Then there is breastfeeding, the opportunity for the mother to bestow on the baby the most blissful of all gifts. Quoting from a number of studies, Ashley Montagu points out that children who are breastfed are physically and mentally superior to the bottlefed, and that this superiority is proportional to the amount of time they have been fed; and that as they grow up, they have a greater ability to love, work, play, and use their minds critically. "What better comfort, what greater reassurance and promise of good things to come can there be for the baby than being held in its mother's arms and put to nurse at her breast?" Most important, the baby at this time learns happiness. If he experiences happiness truly and deeply, he will know that happiness is possible. He will be able to feel it, conceive it, transmit it to others.

At this time the baby also begins to learn to relate to others. Aldous Huxley wrote in *Island* about a practical and direct way in which, at this time, love can be taught as a concrete reality, rather than just a word or concept:

> Stroke the baby while you are feeding him, it doubles his pleasure. Then, while he is sucking and being caressed, introduce him to the animal or person you want him to love. Rub his body against theirs; let there be a warm physical contact between child and love object. At the same time repeat some word like "good." At first he will understand only the tone of your voice. Later on, when he learns to speak, he will get the full meaning. Food plus caress plus contact plus "good" equals love. And love equals pleasure, love equals satisfaction.

Holding, caressing and rocking, together with breastfeeding, the hold the key for a successful caring development. Recent research shows that lack of physical stimulation in the early months of life brings about a condition known as "anedonia," the inability to experience pleasure. James Prescott wrote: "During formative periods of brain growth, certain kinds of sensory deprivation—such as lack of touching and rocking by the mother—result in complete or damaged development of the neuronal systems that control pleasure . . . Since the same systems influence brain centers associated with violence, in a mutually inhibiting mechanism, the deprived infant may have difficulty controlling violent impulses as an adult."

Science finds it easier to measure visible pathologies. You will probably experience more pleasure in imagining both the visible and invisible benefits that a close early contact with the baby can bring about. You can time travel far into the future. Imagine him as a grown-up—a healthy, happy person with strength and vitality vibrating in his whole being; with the joy of living radiating all around him and reaching out, as a blessing; with that centeredness and that maturity which no stress can destroy; and with a facility to relate with others, understand them, please them, without having to depend on them.

If the message in this chapter had to be summed up, one word would do: empathy. Empathy enables us to identify with other human beings, feel their feelings and sensation, see the world from their point of view, be them. Without it, we become isolated robots, troubled and troublemakers. Prisoners of our own universe, we feel poor and lonely.

But the barriers of our egos can be loosened. With the help of our imagination, we can participate in other people's lives, see reality through their eyes, feel their feelings and sense their cravings. Shelley saw in this faculty the making of a poet: "A man, to be greatly good, must imagine intensely and comprehensively; he must put himself in the place of another and of many others; the pains and pleasures of his species must become his own." We all have the ability to empathize when we are children; then, as life's battles and toils harden us, we let it slowly atrophy. We become more and more enclosed in our universe. The world, in turn, responds to us with the same tune, so we forget even more. Fortunately, we can reverse this trend and at least partially recover our forgotten gift.

Become a Baby Again

The following meditation will be a step toward re-awakening or enhancing your capacity for empathy. Life will provide plenty of other occasions, with your baby and with others, for continuing this work.

Lie down, close your eyes, breathe deeply and easily. Gradually, without hurry, you feel that each breath takes you closer and closer to being a baby, perhaps your baby. As you go further back in time, you leave all the familiar structures, habits, environments, ideas, that you have gradually built around yourself or become accustomed to during these years. This is a journey to simplicity, to the unadulterated innocence of infancy.

Now is the time to be a little baby again, feel how it feels to have—

> *. . . no ability to structure or categorize what you see,*

> *. . . an overwhelming need for closeness and touch,*

> *. . . a wordless vulnerability,*

> *. . . a bundle of intense, yet diffused bodily sensations,*

> *. . . an absolute openness to relation,*

> *. . . a skin so amazingly delicate.*

Now is the time for you to be a baby again . . . take a long time in doing so, and imagine yourself to be in a variety of situations.

Now is the time to experience being left suddenly alone in the dark, to have the emptiness and the cold of uninhabited space around you, moving your arms and hands, and wanting to reach, and finding no one.

Now is the time to imagine, as a baby, what it feels like to be surrounded by the cold, glaring impersonality of neon lights:

. . . to be jarred by the harsh sounds of television;

. . . to have rough textures on your skin, the touch of unfeeling hands, hurrying to do their job or clothing that constrains you;

. . . to reel with impotent rage for not being understood at all when your well-being and—you feel—your survival are at stake.

Now, now is the time for you to feel what it is to be left utterly, completely, desperately alone.

Again, breathe deeply and slowly for a while. Now, as a baby still, you feel rocked with a pleasant, regular rhythm:

. . . you feel the bliss of plunging your face in the warmth of welcoming breasts;

. . . the heavenly sweetness of milk;

. . . the wonderful security of being embraced by protective arms;

. . . the comfort of seeing loving eyes looking at you;

. . . the happiness of receiving that mysterious, volatile, infinitely precious substance that only your mother's smile can transmit.

Open your eyes again, then make drawings of what you felt and needed as a baby or as your baby. Remember, as always, whether you know or not how to draw does not matter in the least now.

Still expressing the baby's viewpoint, write a letter to someone who understands you. Say all that

*you have experienced, and all that you have
needed.*

It will be highly beneficial for the baby if you can
experience even vaguely what he experiences; and it will be
profoundly refreshing and useful for you as well. However, this
meditation is just an example of how you can develop your
powers of empathy with your baby.

This child of your dreams will be your best teacher, if you
are ready to receive his teaching. He will be your greatest love,
if you are willing to receive his tenderness. He will be the most
amusing clown, if you are ready to have fun with him. At times
this child may also be the most difficult challenge, demanding all
the patience you will be able to muster. Finally, he will be your
creation, and a very special one: a creation that detaches itself
from the creator, unfolds, and acquires a life of its own, endlessly
surprising. And you are the one who started and nourished this
person into becoming what he or she is meant to be.

With the warmth and the strength of your thoughts, you
have facilitated the unfolding, you will have made a dream come
true. Coleridge said: "Imagine that you dream of Heaven, and
on Heaven you find a wonderful flower, and the next morning,
on awakening, you find that same flower of your dreams by you
. . ." This is our wish to you, that the most beautiful dreams you
have dreamed shall come true. Thus the Great Story will
continue, a story in which so many different events are
represented, so many colors used. And the threads which make
it up are precious threads of love.

Project Caressing

An infant crying in the night:
An infant crying for the light:
And with no language but a cry.
         —Tennyson

It is at the two extremes of life that loneliness is most acutely felt. The baby that is not fondled and caressed in its first two years of life will become neurotic, miasmic, unresponsive, delinquent, or underachieving—the problem being determined by genes or culture. Each of these afflictions generates isolation and loneliness.

At the other end of the spectrum older people, still young in body and spirit, are obliged to retire professionally, find themselves alienated from their families, and often have to give up their homes. All these people can look forward to one beautiful opportunity offered: caressing.

For Project Caressing we envision in every city block a serene, soundproof, pastel-colored room, furnished only with comfortable rocking armchairs and pillows. The adult participants give an hour or more of their time to hold a baby, knowing that their warmth and affection will magically infuse the child's entire life with responsive tenderness. No words will interfere with the soft melting of loneliness into silent loving communication—only soothing humming in the "Caressing Room," or golden silence. For in the world of the infant, it is the contact with a living body and with a beating heart that counts. The busy mothers and fathers will be able to leave the infant in the "Caressing Room," knowing that only affection and tranquillity will be there, rather than the catastrophic noises, lights, and radiations of television, so often used as a built-in, never quiet, never caring babysitter. The older people, who more and more are becoming separated from their grandchildren, will feel the joy of giving—not money or work or material things—but giving themselves and their love for the sheer pleasure of it. They will hold a baby, feel its pure tender skin, and by the magic of touching they will be touched.

Project Caressing is an on-going project of Our Ultimate Investment. There are several Caressing Rooms in Los Angeles, and there is a great demand for more throughout the country. You too may want to open a Caressing Room in your own city. For information, write to OUI, 6301 Sunset Blvd., Suite 103, Los Angeles, CA 90028.

Facts You Should Know

The objective, factual attitude of science has been applied to the most intimate of relationships. The ineffable has been scrutinized in the smallest detail. The graceful union of man and woman has been examined with the cold objectivity of experimental research. Should we consider it a violation? Not in the least! On the contrary, the scientific approach has made our understanding more complete and compassionate.

1. More than half of the six million pregnancies taking place each year in America are unintended. Nearly half of these are terminated by abortion. ["Half Our Pregnancies Are Unintentional," *Newsweek*, October 10, 1983, 37.]

2. It is easiest to study the results of unwanted pregnancy by studying the children born after their mothers had requested abortion—and the request had been denied. In a study conducted on 220 children born of Czechoslovakian mothers who have been denied abortion, it was found that they had more difficulty adjusting socially and were more prone than others to acute illness and hospitalization. In a similar study conducted in Sweden, children born unwanted received twice as much psychiatric help, received more public assistance between the ages of sixteen and twenty-one, showed a higher rate of delinquency, and got less education. [J. Segal, *A Child's Journey* (New York: McGraw-Hill, 1978), 54-55.]

3. Among the many causes of delinquency, unwanted pregnancy is a major one. In a study conducted on the early developmental history of 136 delinquents, most conditions were found to be average or better than average: the overwhelming majority of the mothers had been in good health during pregnancy, most deliveries and the babies' development had been normal, breastfeeding had been prolonged. One factor only differentiated the delinquents: 84% of them, according to their mothers, were unwanted. [W. C. Kvaraceus, "Prenatal and Early Developmental History of 136 Delinquents," *Journal of Genetic Psychology*, 66 (1945): 267-71.]

4. In this country 96 out of 1000 girls and young women between the ages of 15 and 19 become pregnant, four-fifths of them by mistake; and 40% of all girls who are 14 years old now will be pregnant at least once by the time they are 20. [Research of the Alan Guttmacher Institute, New York, 1985.]

5. The above situation is self-perpetuating: 82% of girls who give birth at age 15 or younger were daughters of teenage mothers. ["Children Having Children," *Time*, December 9, 1985, 79.]

6. Although at first teenage fathers are eager to help and maintain contact with their babies, after a year or so the financial contributions drop and the fathers begin to disappear. [Bryan E. Robinson and Robert L. Barret, "Teenage Fathers," *Psychology Today*, December 1985, 68.]

7. Two percent of children born to parents younger than 17 die before completing their first year (twice the rate of other babies). This is attributed to the immaturity of the parents and the lack of appropriate care. Teenage parents are also statistically more likely to abuse their children. [Bryan E. Robinson and Robert L. Barret, "Teenage Fathers," *Psychology Today*, December 1985, 70.]

8. Estimates of the actual number of child abuse incidents range between one and two million per year. About 2000 children die each year under circumstances that suggest child abuse. [*Phi Delta Kappan*, February 1985, 435-6.]

9. The families of abused children are mainly composed of female-headed households, receive public assistance, have younger caretakers, and are subject to economic hardships. [*Trends in Child Abuse and Neglect: A National Perspective*, published in 1985 by the Children's National Division of the American Humane Association.]

10. Smoking in either parent before conception increases the possibility of having a deformed child. It can cause genetic mutation which is then transmitted through the generations. Ultimately, it contributes to changing the genetic pool of humanity. [Stewart Brand, "Human Harm to Human DNA," *Coevolution Quarterly*, no. 21 (Spring 1979): 9, 18.]

11. Smoking in the pregnant mother may cause premature birth, low birth weight, increased risk of miscarriage, learning and memory deficits in the developing fetus. ["Pre-birth Co Linked to Learning Defects," *Science News*, 125, no. 22, June 2, 1984, 348.]

12. In research carried out by the National Institute of Child Health and Human Development in Bethesda, more than 30,000 women were asked about their drinking habits during pregnancy. The results: the more a mother drank, the more she was likely to have an underweight baby—an indicator of a poor state of health in the baby. In another study, conducted by the University of Washington in Seattle, it was found that eight months after birth this damage had remained. [Jody Gaylin, "Childbirth News," *New York*, February 11, 1985, 62.]

13. Through the ordinary sounds of everyday living, events of the mother's life write their story deeply in the fetus's

dawning psyche. San Francisco therapist Jack Downing had a client who suffered from the intense pain of his father's rejection. The client relived a painful prenatal memory in which his mother announced her pregnancy to his father. The father, upset because he had been saving to buy a Chrysler, wanted her to have an abortion. The two fought bitterly, then never again discussed the matter (when Downing's client questioned his parents about the incident, they reluctantly acknowledged it). This catharsis brought about a decisive improvement in the client's outlook and will to live. Thus, the prenatal memory of an argument long past had survived in him as a blurred but intense and all-encompassing hurt. Many therapists related similar incidents. ["Pre-birth Memories Appear to Have Lasting Effect," *Brain-Mind Bulletin*, February 15, 1982, 1.]

14. Fetuses can differentiate and remember the sounds of words. Sixteen mothers were asked to read aloud the story *The Cat in the Hat* by Dr. Seuss to their fetuses twice a day, during the last six and a half weeks of pregnancy. When the babies were born, they were made to hear a tape or their mother reading *The Cat in the Hat*, and also another story, *The King, The Mice and the Cheese*. All the babies showed signs of preferring *The Cat in the Hat*. (The baby can clearly signal its preferences by the way and patterns of sucking.) [Gina Kolata, "Studying Learning in the Womb," *Science*, July 20, 1984, 303.]

15. The National Academy of Sciences recommends a weight increase of 25 to 30 pounds for the pregnant woman. If the mother restricts her calorie intake during pregnancy, this may result in undernourishment for the unborn child. [Judy Willis, "All About Eating for Two," *FDA Consumer*, March 6, 1984, 9.]

16. According to researchers in Lyon, France, the pregnant woman metabolizes caffeine in a way that is different from the

nonpregnant woman: she is half as slow to eliminate it from her body. The caffeine easily crosses the placenta, and the fetus is even slower in dealing with it. Thus poisonous levels of caffeine may accumulate around the fetus. ["Pregnancy Is No Time for Major Stress," *Prevention*, December 1984, 153.]

17. Should there be full sexual intercourse during pregnancy? Some research suggests that a great amount of caution needs to be taken. A Herschey Medical Center study of 27,000 newborns indicated that there is an increased possibility of death, respiratory distress, and jaundice in the babies whose mothers and fathers have intercourse during the last months of pregnancy. [*Today's Child*, January 1980, 6.]

18. Women who go through labor without anesthesia suffer more pain than anesthetized women do, but also experience more pleasure and have a more beautiful recollection of childbirth, according to research conducted at the Queen Charlotte's Maternity Hospital in London. [Virginia Adams, "Pain and Pleasure in Childbirth," *Psychology Today*, March 1983, 71.]

19. In an eleven-year research project on death following cesarean section in Rhode Island, it was found that risk of death from cesarean section was 26 times greater than with vaginal delivery. [Nancy Wainer Cohen and Lois J. Estner, "Silent Knife: Cesarean Section in the United States," *Society*, 21, no. 1 (November-December, 1983): 106.]

20. Drs. Brackbill and Broman found, in studying the data from 3,500 healthy women, that medication at the time of delivery affects the child's behavior at least through seven years of age. According to Dr. Brackbill, the average I.Q. loss per medicated birth is four points—which means 14,060,000 IQ points lost to new U.S. citizens every year. [Diana Korte and Roberta Scaer, *A Good Birth, A Safe Birth* (New York: Bantam Books, 1984).]

21. In Holland, about 50% of the women have their babies in the hospital and 50% have them at home. The mortality-morbidity rates are one-third lower at home than they are in the hospitals. [Ashley Montagu, OUI Conference, 1978.]

22. According to Russian researcher Igor Tjarkovsky the newborn should find a situation similar to the one he had in the womb—namely, weightlessness and a liquid environment. With his help, mothers deliver their babies in the water.

In the water, babies feel freer, more at ease. It is their natural element, and they don't need to make any effort to get used to it. In fact, fear of water is a learned response, and "water babies" who are not affected by it, show a great confidence with the liquid domain. Very soon they breastfeed, move, play and dance underwater with ease and delight. They look free and strong when they are a few weeks old, and seem to belong to another and more advanced phase in our evolution.

This is not only an impression. While in normal births the adjustment calls for extraordinary expenditure of energy for the baby, no such effort is required in water birth. All the extra energy which is liberated benefits the whole organism. Tjarkovsky found that babies born in this way are calmer, more independent, more intelligent and harmonious than the ones born in traditional settings.

The water birth approach is starting to be used in the West too. Dr. Odent found that it makes life easier for the mother: in the water mothers lose their inhibitions and tensions faster, delivery is quicker and easier, pain is lessened, and risk is not increased. [Eric Sidenbladh, *Water Babies: The Igor Tjarkovsky Method for Delivery in Water* (New York: St. Martin's Press, 1983).]

23. In a study involving 49 cultures, Prescott found that when the levels of affection with babies are low, the levels of violence in the adults are high, and when the levels of affection

with the babies are high, the levels of violence in the adults are low. He convincingly linked the lack of affection in the early years with sexual crimes, alcoholism, drug abuse, high divorce rates, depressive and autistic behavior, hyperactivity, and emotional disturbances. He also found that deprivation of affection and physical contact in the early years is compensated during adolescence with a frantic search for unqualified body pleasure and immediate gratification. [James W. Prescott, "Alienation of Affection," *Psychology Today*, December 1979, 124.]

24. Recent studies at U.C. Berkeley, the University of Illinois, and in Japan show that pregnant rats placed in an enriched environment—with novel and constantly varied toys, ladders, and tubes—give birth to rats with larger brains and superior maze-learning skills. There is also good evidence that the observed changes in the brain anatomy of "enriched rats," including a thickened cortex, are permanent. These findings support the 2000-year-old Japanese tradition, *taikyo*, which posits that "enriching the mother's experience . . . influences the unborn child's future intelligence." ["Mother's Enriched Environment Alters Brains of Unborn Rats," "Maternal-Enrichment Studies Support Ancient Oriental Tradition," *Brain-Mind Bulletin*, March 1987, 1, 4-5.]

25. In a pilot project of Our Ultimate Investment we brought together ten 9- to 15-year-old boys and girls from various schools and different social backgrounds. They were invited to be with children aged from one to five and earn academic credit for their time. Three times a week, boys and girls interacted freely with toddlers, under the supervision of three high school teachers at a primary school bearing the promising name of First Step, in Santa Monica, California. At the end of two hours, after the parents fetched the toddlers, we held a seminar with discussion among the students, the coordinators, and at times other participants. The students discussed freely

their feelings and reactions to the experience. The atmosphere was informal, with no attempt made to instruct, persuade, or manipulate in any way the students' responses.

At the end of a six-week period we made a general evaluation. The reactions were alike and significant. Generally the young students were surprised to learn how demanding it is to be with a child, how one's attention is constrained and energy is soon spent—and all that during only two hours! Students compared this with the parents' 24 hours every day. Some students were embarrassed when faced with beings bubbling with strength, desires and feelings of their own. Other students experienced a reawakening of the child within them—the infants they had been in their own development, and were already forgetting. Many of the students reached the conclusion that they would wait until they were twenty-eight or thirty before having children—if ever. They were overwhelmed by the powerful, almost implacable demands of the toddlers. They saw how the infants' natural self-centeredness would impinge on the time and space a young adult needs for his own interests and development.

Suggested Reading

Arms, Suzanne, *Immaculate Deception*. New York: Bantam Books, 1984.

Bradley, Robert A., M.D., *Husband–Coached Childbirth*. New York: Harper & Row, 1974.

Dick-Read, Grantly, M.D., *Childbirth Without Fear*, 2nd ed. New York: Harper & Brothers, 1959.

Huxley, Aldous, *Island*. New York: Harper & Brothers, 1962.

Klause, M.H., and Kennell, J.H., *Maternal-Infant Bonding*. St. Louis: Mosby, 1976.

Korte, Diana, and Scaer, Roberta, *A Good Birth, A Safe Birth*. New York: Bantam Books, 1984.

Liley, Albert W., "The Foetus as Personality." *Child and Family* 11, No. 3 (1972): 225.

Montagu, Ashley, *Life Before Birth*. New York: Signet, 1978.

Mothering, journal published by Mothering Publications, P.O. Box 8410, Santa Fe, New Mexico, 87054.

Nilsson, Lennart, *A Child Is Born*. New York: Dell Publishing Co., 1986.

Odent, Michel, *Birth Reborn*. New York: Pantheon Books, 1984.

Schwartx, Leni, *The World of the Unborn*. New York: Richard Marek Publishers, 1980.

Sidenbladh, Erik, *Water Babies: The Igor Tjarkovsky Method for Delivery in Water*. New York: St. Martin's Press, 1983.

Verny, Thomas, and Kelly, John, *The Secret Life of the Unborn Child*. New York: Delta Publishing Co., 1986.

Prayer of the Unconceived

Men and women who are on Earth
You are our creators.
We, the unconceived, beseech you:
Let us have living bread
The builder of our new body.
Let us have pure water
The vitalizer of our blood.
Let us have clean air
So that every breath is a caress.
Let us feel the petals of jasmine and roses
Which are as tender as our skin.

Men and women who are on Earth
You are our creators.
We, the unconceived, beseech you:
Do not give us a world of rage and fear
For our minds will be rage and fear.
Do not give us violence and pollution
For our bodies will be disease and abomination.
Let us be wherever we are
Rather than bringing us
Into a tormented and self-destroying humanity.

Men and women who are on Earth
You are our creators.
We, the unconceived, beseech you:
If you are ready to love and to be loved,
Invite us to this Earth
Of the thousand wonders,
And we will be born
To love and to be loved.